Anorexia Nervosa
A Guide to Recovery

Anorexia Nervosa
A Guide to Recovery

Lindsey Hall
and
Monika Ostroff

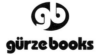

gürze books

Anorexia Nervosa
A Guide to Recovery

© 1999 by Lindsey Hall & Monika Ostroff

Gürze Books
P.O. Box 2238
Carlsbad, CA 92018
(760)434-7533

Cover design by Abacus Graphics, Oceanside, CA
Fabric art by Dorothy Turk

Library of Congress
Cataloging-in-Publication Data

Hall, Lindsey, 1949-
    Anorexia nervosa : a guide to recovery / Lindsey Hall & Monika Ostroff.
        p. cm.
    Includes bibliographical references and index.
    ISBN 0-936077-32-8 (alk. paper)
    1. Anorexia nervosa—Popular works. I. Ostroff, Monika.
    II. Title.
    RC552.A5H35   1998
    616.85'262—dc21   98-29374
                                            CIP

NOTE:
The authors and publisher of this book intend for this publication to provide accurate information. It is sold with the understanding that it is meant to complement, not substitute for, professional medical and/or psychological services.

9   8   7   6   5

Let us all
love and respect
each other
and ourselves.

Table of Contents

Acknowledgments

Many generous people contributed to this book. I am especially grateful to Monika Ostroff for her willingness to work so closely with a person she had never met, and for the depth and compassion of her writing. I also give thanks to my children for their patience and humor; to my assistant, Mary Ann, for giving me the space and time to write; and to my dear friend, Mar, for her support and open heart.

I also appreciate the editing assistance of Dina Wolff and the participation of Leigh Cohn, my husband and the publisher of Gürze Books, who was instrumental in every stage of this project from its inception to publication.

Thanks, as well, to the many anonymous contributors whose voices are such a vital aspect of this book. Sharing with each other gives us strength and hope.

Lindsey Hall

This book has been greatly enriched by many special people. I would like to thank my husband, Sam, for the sparkle he adds to my life and for his unwavering faith in my ability to hold the stars in my hand. I am especially grateful to Sarah, whose patience and continued compassionate support has been such a vital healing force in my life. A special thanks goes to Jeanne Williamson, Josh, Elaine, and Earl Ostroff for the abundance of support that came in so many different forms; and to Barbara Peoples, Lara JK Wilson, and Lisa Goodrich for their enthusiasm, skill, and honesty.

I also greatly appreciate the wisdom and encouragement that came from Therese Zimmer, LCSW; Diane Gibson, RD; Sarah Warren, Psy.D.; Jane MacDonald, Ph.D.; Mona Villapiano, Psy.D.; and John Temte, MD. A heartfelt thank you goes to the many anonymous voices for sharing their perspective, strength and hope.

I would especially like to thank Lindsey Hall and Leigh Cohn for embarking on this project with me with such vision, vitality, and openness.

Thank you to all who have blessed my world with their very special light!

Monika Ostroff

Introduction

This book is for people who want to understand and recover from anorexia nervosa. Both of the authors of this book have fully recovered from eating disorders, and many individuals who have recovered or are recovering from anorexia also contributed insights and suggestions.* Whether you yourself are suffering with anorexia or you know someone who is, their wisdom can inspire and guide you.

As you will read in Chapter 2, Monika Ostroff battled with anorexia for many years. She shares her story of self-starvation, years of unsuccessful treatment, and eventual breakthroughs that led to her complete recovery. Her ideas about the nature of anorexia and what it takes to defeat obsessive food behaviors and thoughts encompass much of the text. She writes with understanding and compassion; and, when she recommends that you try something, it is because it has worked for her.

Lindsey Hall has written several books about recovering from eating disorders, beginning in 1980 when she first wrote her story in a booklet titled, "Eat Without Fear." It was the first publication ever printed about bulimia, and was eventually included in the book, *Bulimia: A Guide to Recovery,* which has helped hundreds of thousands of sufferers, their loved ones, and the professionals

---

* Indicated with *italics* throughout the book.

who treat them. The structure of this book is similar to *Bulimia*, which is now in its fifth edition and has been translated into several languages. Lindsey has devoted her life to eating disorders education and recovery, and her experience as an author, speaker, and pioneer in the field is further detailed in the "About the Authors" section in the back of the book. She shares her expertise with the same love and awareness that has touched so many others who have recovered from eating disorders.

The first chapter of this book answers the most commonly asked questions about anorexia and recovery, including basic facts as well as personal observations. The information will help you to more fully understand that anorexia nervosa is a complex condition with serious physical, emotional, and spiritual consequences.

The next chapter is Monika's inspirational story, "Searching for Safety." Although she had to be hospitalized several times and many doctors gave up on her, Monika did recover from anorexia. She cured herself because of her willingness and courage to try different approaches, the commitment to persevere, and hard work. She eventually teamed up with a therapist who believed in her, which helped Monika believe in herself.

The next six chapters of the book cover specific topics to explore as you begin your recovery process.

Chapter 3 tells you where to start, and Chapter 4 explains why outside support is so important and has suggestions on where to find it. The next chapter is divided into several sections that offer advice based on "What has Worked for Many" people in recovery. Each section addresses one main idea, such as "Journal Writing" or "Be Gentle with Your Pain." Examples, activities, lists of ideas, and quotes from various contributors are also included.

These things-to-do have proven to be successful, and if you try them, you can be, too. Chapter 6 discusses "Healthy Eating and Healthy Weight." It describes how set point and metabolism affect your body, and recommends how to approach your fears about eating and gaining weight. Chapter 7 is on how to stay committed and what to do about ambivalence or relapse.

Chapter 8 is a "Guide for Parents and Loved Ones" which you should read and show to the other important people in your life. It lists basic suggestions, with short explanations to help you all approach your situation with optimism. Resources for you and them are also provided in the last chapter.

Obviously, recovering from an eating disorder requires more than simply reading a self-help book. It requires determination, hard work, and the involvement of others. If you follow the advice that is offered here, you will lead a happier and healthier life. You will learn to love yourself and appreciate the miracle that is your body. You will value your existence in the world and enrich your life with good relationships. All this may not come quickly or easily, but it will absolutely be worthwhile.

CHAPTER 1

Questions
Most Often Asked
About Anorexia Nervosa

What is anorexia nervosa?

Anorexia nervosa, in the most simple terms, is self-starvation. Anorexics (anorectic is also correct usage) are typically described as "walking skeletons," a graphic image that depicts the pallor and frailty of these struggling individuals. Anorexics are also often characterized as stubborn, vain, appearance-obsessed people who simply do not know when to stop dieting. But anorexia nervosa is much more than just a diet gone awry, and the sufferer more than an obstinate, skinny person refusing to eat. It is a complex problem with intricate roots that often begins as a creative and reasonable solution to difficult circumstances, and is thus a way to cope.

Anorexia is Greek word meaning "loss of appetite," which is misleading because only in the late stages of starvation do people in fact lose their appetites. Instead, an intense fear of weight gain leads anorexics to routinely and vehemently deny their hunger.

In order to formally diagnose an individual with anorexia nervosa, clinicians turn to the fourth edition of the American Psychiatric Association's Diagnostic and Statistical Manual of Mental Disorders (DSM-IV, 1994). The DSM-IV lists four criteria that an individual must meet in order to be diagnosed as anorexic, generalized as follows:

A. The individual maintains a body weight that is about 15% below normal for age, height, and body type.

B. The individual has an intense fear of gaining weight or becoming fat, even though they are underweight. Paradoxically, losing weight can make the fear of gaining even worse.

C. The individual has a distorted body image. Some may feel fat all over, others recognize that they are generally thin but see specific body parts (particularly the stomach and thighs) as being too fat. Their self-worth is based on their body size and shape. They deny that their low body weight is serious cause for concern.

D. In women, there is an absence of at least three consecutive menstrual cycles. A woman also meets this criteria if her period occurs only while she is taking a hormone pill (including, but not limited to, oral contraceptives).

The DSM-IV also differentiates between two specific types of anorexia nervosa. "Restricting Type" denotes individuals who lose weight primarily by reducing their overall food intake through dieting, fasting and/or exercising excessively. "Binge-Eating /Purging Type" describes those who regularly binge (consume large amounts of food in short periods of time), and purge through self-induced vomiting, excessive exercise, fasting, the abuse of diuretics, laxatives, and enemas, or any combination of these measures.

Delineating between the two types of anorexia has cleared up the long-standing confusion of diagnosing individuals who meet all of the criteria for anorexia, but who also engage in bingeing and purging. For many years these individuals were either given both the anorexia nervosa and bulimia nervosa diagnoses, or only the bulimia nervosa diagnosis, because bingeing and purging was typically deemed to be bulimic and not anorexic behavior.

In addition to the criteria set forth by the DSM-IV, anorexics develop and adhere to rigid beliefs and rules. Most only permit themselves a limited number of calories each day, usually no more than a few hundred, which is approximately one quarter of what an "average" moderately-active woman would need in order to maintain a healthy body weight. Throughout the course of their day, many anorexics religiously record the number of calories they have consumed, and if the allotted quota is surpassed, whether accidentally or in the course of a binge, they feel overwhelmed by anxiety, anger, frustration, and fear. In an attempt to alleviate this extreme sense of discomfort, many compensate by adding additional exercise to their daily workout, further restricting their food intake over the course of the next several days, or by purging through forced vomiting or laxative abuse.

Anorexics will delay or avoid meals for as long as possible, because while they may be obsessed with thoughts of food, the actual act of eating is frightening. Eating is even more scary if the food choices are made by someone else, such as parents or caregivers. Other family members may also dread mealtimes, when the conflict between the families' concern and helplessness and the child's obsessive behavior often comes to a head.

Most anorexics limit themselves to foods which are low in calories, such as fruits and vegetables. Because eating these foods is unlikely to result in weight gain, the individual considers them to be "safe" and can consume them with less anxiety. Although anorexics may crave higher calorie foods, these are thought to be "dangerous." In the rare instance that they do ingest something "risky," they agonize over what the food is doing to their bodies, plagued by fears of weight gain. The belief that one bite of a forbidden food will add ten pounds is not uncommon.

As a means of governing their meticulous eating behaviors, many anorexics develop rigid rules, such as never allowing their lips to touch the prongs of a fork, cutting food into a specific number of small pieces or shapes, arranging food in precise places on their plates, eating food in a particular order, and chewing each morsel a specific number of times before swallowing. These rules function to distract them from the anguish of what the food may be doing to their bodies, and create the sense of safety required for them to eat at all.

Anorexics also create rules that extend into other areas of their lives. Many develop a closely guarded exercise regimen, which may include precise numbers of hours, miles, or repetitions for burning calories. Most treat their scale like a deity, giving it the power to determine how they feel about the day and themselves. They also weigh-in multiple times each day, perhaps even at specific times.

Who gets anorexia nervosa?

In the preface to her landmark book on anorexia, *The Golden Cage* (1979), Hilde Bruch describes anorexia nervosa as a "disease that selectively befalls the young, rich, and beautiful." For the most, part people still tend to associate anorexia with white, upper-middle class, heterosexual women; but in fact, anorexia knows no social, cultural, economic, gender, racial, or sexual boundaries. It is by no means a selective disease or affliction; in short, anyone can get anorexia.

Anorexia affects between 1% and 5% of the general population when rigid diagnositic criteria are applied (Zerbe 1995, p. 15), and can occur at almost any age and at any time of life. Children as young as seven and adults well into their senior years have been documented (Lask and Bryant-Waugh 1996, p. 18). Approximately 10% of anorexics are male, although many clinicians claim to see an even smaller percentage in their practices (Andersen 1995, p. 177). While it is true that the majority of anorexics are women, it may not be true that they are primarily white women from a particular economic class. There have been few studies on the prevalence of eating disorders in non-white or lower socioeconomic populations.

Actually, social stereotypes may play a large role in the failure of trained clinicians to accurately diagnose eating disorders in minority populations (Thompson 1996, p. 12). For example, a large African-American woman and a thin Asian woman may be overlooked or not assessed for eating disorders simply because their bodies happen to fit the widely-accepted stereotypes of their respective races. In her book, *A Hunger So Wide And So Deep,* Becky Thompson interviewed eighteen African-American, Latina, and white women, both lesbian and heterosexual. Although each of them met the DSM criteria for eating disorders, only two had been accurately diagnosed. In a survey of 600 African-Americans (Pumariega 1994) researchers concluded that these women "are at risk for eating disorders in at least equal proportions to their white counterparts." These studies dispel the myth that only white women have problems with food and eating.

There are many characterizations in the professional literature of the people who are prone to developing anorexia. In his book, *It's Not Your Fault* (1992), Russell Marx describes the potential anorexics as having smooth preadolescent lives, depicting them as fairly successful, model children. He maintains that the girls develop "fragile personalities" and "lack the inner strength necessary to handle loss," which he defines as divorce, the first romantic break up, going off to college, etc. He suggests they have "aged, but not grown up" (pp. 34-35). For some anorexics this may well be an apt description. However, the women depicted in Becky Thompson's book stand in glaring contrast to Marx's. The women in her study were forced to endure traumatic events and found ways to cope with their difficult circumstances—they grew up *before* they aged. These two opposing descriptions are offered to illustrate that neither anorexics nor their lives may be easily characterized, and to remind us that individuals are just that— individual and unique. Thus, among the active and recovered anorexic contributors to this book are:

A 12-year-old from a white, middle-class family, who does well in school, and has lots of hobbies, such as Taekwondo, acting, playing the piano, and reading.

An Hispanic, feminist, purchasing officer studying toward a BSW.

A former high school and college wrestler.

A waitress from a working class family—"not particularly successful, not necessarily a failure, but somewhere in-between."

A 24-year-old male chemistry graduate student.

A university Latin teacher, the youngest of five children, all of whom wrestled with addictive/compulsive behaviors.

An Italian/Portuguese mother of three, who started dieting in the second grade.

A middle child of 13, who writes poetry and wants to do volunteer work with kids, but who has been unable to work for 10 years due to her illness.

An ESL instructor, ex-diver/gymnast on a national level, honors graduate, who came from an alcoholic/addictive home.

A black female from a large, dysfunctional family, who is the Assistant Director of a woman's program.

Why do people become anorexic?

One common misconception is that people become anorexic because they are self-absorbed, vain individuals who place too much importance on their looks. While the culture of thinness in which we live is certainly an influential factor in the development of anorexia, it is by no means the sole cause. In fact, there is no sole cause. Anorexia is a response to a complex mix of cultural, social, familial, psychological, and biological influences unique to each person. The answer to the question "Why?" is an individual one requiring deep introspection on a personal level. Some possibilities are discussed below.

One widely-accepted theory is that people develop anorexia because they seek control over themselves and their lives. Food and weight can be controlled when other aspects of life cannot, and indeed significant events, such as leaving home for the first time, a divorce, or a serious illness are examples of out-of-control situations which can trigger anorexia. Restricting food intake while in the presence of enticing foods, meticulously adhering to arduous rules and regimens, and successfully losing weight while so many others can't, evokes feelings of accomplishment while providing a sense of security. Eventually, though, anorexics feel even less in control as they become imprisoned by behaviors and thought patterns that, despite concerted efforts, they cannot relinquish.

A high percentage of people struggling with anorexia have a history of abuse, neglect, or other traumatic experiences, and develop anorexia as a coping mechanism. In her book, *A Hunger So Wide And So Deep* (1996), Becky Thompson not only discusses sexual and physical trauma and their relationship to eating disorders, but she also illustrates that living in poverty, enduring acculturation, and suffering racial, sexual, religious, or other forms of discrimination are also traumatic events which can be contributing factors.

Anorexia is an effective way to cope with difficult circumstances because it serves to distract the sufferer from the pain. Losing weight provides a concrete goal that requires energy, planning, and effort. The amount of time spent tallying calories, exercising, and thinking about food is time spent not thinking about pain. Also, many anorexics experience a "high" when they are at a low weight because only there do they feel a sense of power and success. In addition to food restriction, bingeing can both numb and bring comfort. Medical theory suggests that the consumption of carbohydrates boosts serotonin levels in the brain, which in turn alleviates feelings of depression. Similarly, the ingestion of sweet or fatty foods tends to increase the level of endorphins, which are the body's natural pain killers (Marx pp. 88-89). Thus, the phrase "food is a drug" may have validity for some people.

For young men and women, anorexia can be a way to handle the confusion of changing societal roles. These days, it is difficult to know whether being a woman means nurturing or assertive, at home or at work, independent or dependent, etc. Also, in spite of economic and political advances, unnaturally thin bodies continue to be used to sell products and life-styles, implying that the "right body" will bring happiness, success, and a better life. Women on the brink of womanhood receive the conflicting message, "You can be whatever you want to be, but you better be thin." Young men, whose roles are also in flux, face similar conflicts about whether they should be at work or at home, sensitive or tough, the breadwinner or bread maker. They, too, are exposed to images of the perfect body type, muscular, fit, and lean—again, not fat. Anorexia can be a way to postpone or avoid the confusion of what it means to be a modern-day man or woman.

Losing weight is also a way for some women to avoid developing into mature sexual beings, in effect to remain in a child's body without the demands of intimacy and responsibility that accompany adulthood. For example, a survivor of sexual abuse might feel unsafe and would logically reason—consciously or unconsciously—that a body which resembles a preadolescent is no longer sexually desirable or appealing. For her, losing weight could well be a means of protecting herself so that she would be less vulnerable to assaults.

Families are often a factor in the development or maintenance of an eating disorder, although it is sometimes difficult to determine whether family dysfunction is a cause or effect. There may be a predisposition to an eating disorder in families with a history of depression or alcoholism, or who impose actual or perceived rules and expectations on the children. An obsession with food and weight can be an effective way to "disappear" from these unhappy family situations, or in contrast, to take the focus away from other problems at home. Some anorexics alleviate their own discomfort by controlling or manipulating those around them. For example, it is not unusual for an anorexic to do all of the shopping and cooking for a household, while starving herself.

Father/child and mother/child relationships are often central to the development of an eating disorder. "Father Hunger" is a term that refers to the emptiness experienced by children whose fathers are physically or emotionally absent, which creates a void in the family structure. For adolescents at the threshold of adult roles, the absence of a father to guide and reassure them can result in an unrealistic body image, food fears, and insecurity about their roles and budding sexuality. (Maine 1991)

Anorexia can also develop in response to mother/child relationships which have been too close. Relationships such as these make it difficult for a son or daughter to grow into their own, separate identity at the appropriate developmental stage. The child may feel somehow responsible for their mother's happiness or may be afraid of leaving her protection to live in what they both perceive of as a hostile outside world. Mothers sometimes have trouble letting go, as well, when their identity is based on being needed. In many of these cases, anorexia symbolizes an attempt by the child to become an autonomous individual, with boundaries strong enough to keep out intrusion.

Also, family members who diet or make derogatory remarks about fat people clearly deliver the message that thinness is important. In some such cases, anorexia can be the result of dieting competitions between family members, or a way for one member, who is otherwise ignored, to be seen and heard. Losing weight makes them feel powerful and special, providing them with a sense of worth that may otherwise be absent. It is often said that an eating disorder is a way of saying something with the body that cannot be said in words, and this is especially true in families where lines of communication are not always open.

Dieting has become an unfortunate cultural phenomenon, especially for women and girls, whose self image is often closely linked with their body image. Depending on the particular diet, foods are categorized as either "good" or "bad" and they become good or bad for eating them. Sometimes, all it takes is one critical comment from a significant person such as a coach, parent, or friend to begin restricting behaviors. Under the right circumstances, such as those previously mentioned, dieting can easily become an illness.

Unfortunately, the message that thinner is better is affecting younger and younger children. One study of fourth grade girls reports that 80% had already dieted. Many young girls are unaware that they will naturally gain weight during puberty, and begin to restrict their food intake at a time when nature is preparing them for childbirth and they especially need to grow. For many, dieting is disguised as healthy eating, as when a vegetarian diet is manipulated to include only apples and oranges, or when an eating plan includes little or no fat at all. All too often, even when their weight drops below a certain point, many girls have trouble seeing their bodies realistically and insist that they are still fat.

Individuals with anorexia are often described as having been model children who have always done what was expected of them. This has a flip side, for in putting the needs of others first, these children do not develop an adequate sense of self. This low self-esteem can underlie other characteristics such as perfectionism, denial of one's own needs, and approval seeking, all of which are integral symptoms of anorexia. This desire to please, combined with onset of sexual development and the persuasiveness of cultural values, puts teenagers at particular risk.

It is important to remember that different people develop anorexia for different reasons, and what may be true for one person may not be for another. Whatever the reasons, they deserve to be heard, respected, explored, and addressed.

Here are some of the causes that our contributors gave for their eating disorders:

My childhood was very scary and pain-filled. Anorexia helped me to be unaware of my feelings, wants, and needs in order to survive.

Food problems isolated me from myself and others. Focusing on food and weight kept me from seeing how horrible my home life really was.

Focusing on my body has helped me to avoid more pressing problems, such as the sadness of the declining health of loved ones, marital/parental conflicts, and feelings of failure.

My father's emotional abuse clearly contributed to my illness. I have now distanced myself emotionally from my family of origin. This has been painful, but necessary. My recovery depended upon my refusing to continue to tolerate unacceptable behavior.

I used anorexia to hide from the real issues like relationship problems, low self-esteem, loneliness, and shyness.

Thinness brings confidence, attention, activity. To my anorexic self, thin was the answer to all my problems. Thin gave me that

*which I craved most—attention. My anorexic self was unable to
see that thin brought a false confidence and it was the confidence
(not the thinness) that led to friendships, dates, etc.*

How do I know if I have an eating disorder?

This is a difficult question to answer because only you know
the degree to which your preoccupation is interfering with your
life. However, if you answer "yes" to any of the questions below,
whether you fit the DSM-IV criteria for anorexia, bulimia, or another clinically diagnosed disorder, food and weight may be a
problem for you that needs to be addressed. Respond honestly:

DO YOU HAVE AN EATING DISORDER?

- Does the description in the section "What is Anorexia Ner-
  vosa?" describe you?
- Are you constantly thinking about food?
- Is it difficult to concentrate on the daily tasks of studying or
  work because of food and weight thoughts?
- Do you worry about what your last meal is doing to your
  body?
- Do you experience guilt or shame around eating?
- Is it difficult for you to eat in public?
- Do you count calories every time you eat or drink?
- When others tell you that you are too thin, do you still feel fat?
- If you see yourself as thin, do you still obsess about your
  stomach, hips, thighs, or buttocks being too big?
- Do you weigh yourself several times daily?

- Does the number on your scale determine your mood and outlook for the day?
- When you are momentarily satisfied with your weight, do you resolve to be even more vigilant?
- Do you punish yourself with more exercise or restrictions if you don't like the number on the scale?
- Do you exercise more than forty-five minutes, five times each week with the goal of burning calories?
- Will you exercise to lose weight even if you are ill or injured?
- Do you label foods as "good" and "bad?"
- If you eat a "bad" or forbidden food do you berate yourself and compensate by skipping your next meal, purging, or adding extra exercise?
- Do you vomit after eating and/or use laxatives or diuretics to keep your weight down?
- Do you severely limit your food intake?

A professional familiar with the treatment of eating disorders can give you honest feedback about the seriousness of your situation as well as advice about what you may want to do next. Certainly, sharing your thoughts, concerns, and feelings with someone who can listen compassionately while suspending judgment can be helpful and comforting, even motivating. But if you are not ready to change your behaviors, you at least deserve help maintaining your physical and medical safety, something a professional with experience treating anorexia can do for you.

I was called fat names in my gymnastics class and weight became a big issue. I was crushed inside. I didn't know then that this would lead to years of psychological and physical pain.

My recent marriage forced me to look at my ongoing struggle with food. I felt I didn't have a problem even though I was using food as a distancing mechanism. How easy it is to fool ourselves in today's society!

I was on a strict "diet" for ten years when I finally realized that my life was not my own. I am now in treatment for anorexia.

Is anorexia nervosa dangerous?

Definitely. Anorexia nervosa has a multitude of medical complications ranging from mild to severe. In fact, it is believed that 5-20% of anorexics die, usually from complications associated with self-starvation, such as: heart, kidney, or multiple organ failure, or illnesses like pneumonia, which may be due to an inability to fight infection—all ultimately due to the anorexia. Studies show that the longer one has anorexia, the higher the mortality rate. Someone who has been anorexic for five years has about a 5% chance of mortality, but the rate increases to 18% in individuals who suffer chronically for 30 years (Zerbe p. 250).

Let's take a closer look at some of the complications that can arise during the course of anorexia:

Cardiac Problems

Starving, bingeing, and purging all lead to electrolyte imbalances. Electrolytes, which are chemicals like sodium, potassium, and chloride, help regulate heart beat. When dehydration occurs, electrolytes such as potassium are lowered, which may result in cardiac arrhythmia, an irregular heart beat—too fast, too slow, or lacking the proper rhythm. While it is true that some arrhythmia are not dangerous and may even subside once the body is restored to health, others are extremely dangerous and can lead to cardiac arrest. Like Russian Roulette, there are no guarantees as to who develops an arrhythmia or other severe consequence.

In addition to affecting the heart's rhythm, anorexia can affect its size. When people starve and lose weight, they do not lose only fat, they also lose muscle mass. Since the heart itself is a muscle, starvation can lead to decreases in both mass and chamber size.

Also, in order for the heart to beat, lungs to work, and blood to travel through our veins, the body requires energy. Starving causes an energy crisis, in response to which the body literally slows down to conserve what little energy it has left in order to perform the basic functions required to sustain life. In addition to the metabolism slowing down, the heart rate also slows down, a condition called "bradycardia." Most women's hearts average approximately 80 beats per minute, but some anorexics have had heart rates as low as 25 beats per minute (Kaplan 1993, p. 73).

Gastrointestinal disorders

One of the most common problems experienced by those struggling with anorexia is delayed gastric emptying, which essentially means that food leaves the stomach slower than it would if the body were healthy. Many anorexics complain that they feel unduly bloated and "stuffed" after consuming only a modest meal, some feel full after only a few bites. While this discomfort is founded in a real physical condition, it does tend to subside once eating is normalized.

Anorexics who vomit are at risk for internal bleeding, ulcers, and gastritis, a painful inflammation of the stomach lining. Vomiting can cause a painful swelling of the esophagus, and places undue stress on the stomach, both of which are at risk of rupturing, a condition which is fatal unless immediate medical attention is available. Vomiting also causes enlarged salivary glands sometimes described as "chipmunk cheeks," loss of the gag reflex, and has been linked to the development of hiatal hernias.

Constipation is a common condition resulting from inadequate fiber and food intake. Some individuals have such reduced intestinal motility that medical attention is required. Laxative abuse and overly aggressive refeeding both pose a risk for bowel perforations, which may call for surgical intervention. The small intestine also frequently becomes ineffective in absorbing nutrients and minerals.

MORE RISKS AND COMPLICATIONS

- amenorrhea—due to decreased estrogen production, which causes females to cease ovulation and menstruation

- anemia—a blood disorder characterized by either a decrease in the number of red cells, or a reduction in hemoglobin; the body's ability to carry oxygen from the lungs to its tissues is reduced; often caused by an iron deficiency

- bingeing—an effect of starvation

- bruising

- decreased testicular function—some studies reveal a decrease in testosterone and certain male hormones

- dental decay and discoloration

- depressed immune system
- dizziness
- dry skin; brittle hair and nails
- edema—water retention, most commonly in the ankles and feet
- endocrine abnormalities
- fainting
- high cholesterol—an effect of starvation, not necessarily warranting a low cholesterol diet
- hyperactivity
- hypoglycemia
- increased risk of osteoporosis—bones lose density and fracture easily
- insomnia
- ketosis—the excessive accumulation of ketone bodies in the blood and urine, which is indicative of the body digesting its fat stores as a sole source of energy
- kidney damage/failure—usually due to dehydration; may be worsened by the use of diuretics
- lanugo—the growth of fine hair on the body, which is the body's attempt to keep itself warm when fat stores are depleted
- liver damage—a condition that is usually irreparable
- loss of hair on the head
- low blood pressure

- low body temperature—causes anorexics to feel cold

- muscle cramps and weakness—usually due to electrolyte imbalances

- pancreatitis—the painful swelling of the pancreas evidenced by severe abdominal pain, distention, and fever

- sensitivity to light and sound

- yellow skin—also called hypercarotinemia

My husband lost 50 pounds in six months. Most people think he's dying of something and don't suspect anorexia because it is mostly a woman's disease. Recently I've noticed that he is knocking into walls and is extremely tired. I am very worried.

I was in and out of emergency rooms for dehydration a half-dozen times before an intern ever said the words, "anorexia nervosa." Usually, I'd get an IV for a while and they'd send me home, which allowed me to stay in denial about my real illness.

I got dizzy and even fainted a couple of times. I told my parents it was the flu, but they took it as a sign to get me into treatment.

What thoughts and feelings are associated with anorexia?

Anorexia colors one's entire experience of living, not only ravaging the body but the mind and spirit, as well. Although dieting behaviors might have begun as a way to gain self-esteem and mastery, they escalate into a prison of painful thoughts and confused emotions.

Most notably, anorexics are intensely preoccupied with food; they can't stop thinking about it. However, a preoccupation with food has been shown to be one of the effects of starvation, as documented in a well-known study conducted by Ancel Keys (1950) and his colleagues at the University of Minnesota. These researchers took 36 healthy, psychologically-normal males and cut their food intake in half, causing them to lose about 25% of their body weight. Keys studied the men's behavior for a six-month period of food restriction and for three months of rehabilitation. This imposed starvation caused bingeing, food preoccupation, poor judgement, lack of concentration, depression, anxiety, irritability, social withdrawal and lower self-esteem—all symptoms of anorexia.

This study makes clear the importance of weight gain for successful recovery, because of the mental and emotional disabilities associated with weight loss. Sufferers cannot think clearly enough to make proper decisions, problem-solve, or reap the full benefits of therapy. They are trapped in harmful thought patterns, such as "black and white" thinking, where everything is divided into extreme categories. For example, foods are labeled either "good" or "bad," bodies are either "fat" or "thin," and not being completely in-control means being completely out-of-control. There is no middle ground. Other examples of negative thought patterns are magnifying problems, magical thinking, and taking remarks or situations too personally.

These distorted, habitual thinking patterns are rooted in deeply-held belief systems, which make change extremely difficult.

Anorexics typically believe that they can only be happy if they are thin, and that self-indulgence is a sign of weakness. Most devastating of all is the underlying belief in their own worthlessness, which is inextricably tied to the size of their bodies. "I am fat and fat is bad," or, "I am bad if I eat." These deeply-held beliefs make it possible for individuals with anorexia to deny their real needs for nourishment and self-nurturing. They may *think* of themselves as more pure, cleaner, and healthier by not eating, but in reality they are starving their bodies and their souls.

Not only are thought patterns affected by starvation, but feelings are affected as well. One common assumption is that anorexia numbs emotions, but this is not entirely true. It is probably more accurate to say that an eating disorder is a distraction from certain emotions by diverting them into food and weight-related rituals. Painful or unacceptable feelings are translated into feelings having to do with food and the body. For example, what appears to be an intense fear of fat or need for control is hiding deeper feelings, such as anger, rejection, or depression.

Many of the ways that we handle our feelings are learned at an early age. Children who grow up in families where their emotional needs are not met do not have the opportunity to express the normal feelings of growing up. Some families don't want to deal with negative emotions, such as anger or disappointment, and kids learn to monitor or repress their emotions. An anorexic who has not had experience identifying and talking about her feelings will not be able to pinpoint exactly what she is feeling, or she might assume that her feelings are bad and that she is bad for having them.

Anorexia serves as a way to keep feelings at bay. Unfortunately, this illness comes with its own share of shame, loneliness, and fears which are then layered over the original negative feelings. The artificial high that comes from losing weight turns into fear of losing that control and possibly embarrassment.

Even the feeling of success that accompanies the superhuman willpower to not eat is tempered with self-doubt. Anorexics can never be thin enough or as good at doing anything other than losing weight. Sometimes, other people complicate this issue by complementing them on their thinness by saying such things as, "You look great, I wish I could lose weight like you can." Recovering anorexics must learn that this type of response is typical in a culture that values thinness to such a degree, and that success is not measured by external standards, such as the size of one's body. Real success is based on how one thinks and feels on the inside. Everyone acknowledges that their thoughts and feelings change dramatically in recovery, becoming more positive, joyous, meaningful, and empowering.

I became very unhappy, angry, lost all motivation and sense of purpose in life. I was distant to reality, and lived in a different world. When I first started therapy I couldn't even imagine any other life than the unhappy, self-hating one I was living.

It was difficult for me to concentrate on much of anything. My mind wandered in classes and it took me about three times longer than it should have to turn out any kind of quality work. I look back on the energy that went into counting calories and thinking about food, and I feel sad. It was such a shallow and lonely existence.

Anorexia masked my feelings so well that I didn't always recognize them. Back then I couldn't deal with any kind of anger, but now I'm slowly learning to accept it as a part of me.

Recovery reconnected me to my true emotions. They feel much more intense, and somehow more real. I feel more real. I have so much hope and a zest for life that I never thought I could have!

What role does exercise play?

Most anorexics consider exercise to be their best friend because it is a valuable asset in their pursuit of thinness. For someone who consumes too few calories, though, exercise keeps the body in a continual state of deprivation and actually serves as a method of purging. Exercise releases the individual from feelings of guilt and self-blame associated with indulgence—the more food that is eaten, the more rigorous the exercise regime. It is a form of self-control, a way to deny the body's need for rest, and the soul's need to come to grips with what is lacking in their lives.

Compulsive exercise, also referred to as "obligatory exercise" or "activity anorexia" is a common symptom of anorexia. In addition to traditional forms of exercise, like running or playing sports, anorexics seem to be in perpetual motion, running up and down stairs, doing sit ups in the middle of the night, even swinging their legs or bouncing their knees while sitting.

Many anorexics exercise to such a degree that there is little time left for friends, family, school, work, and other aspects of life. Some experience feelings of superiority from being able to exercise more than other people, in the same way that losing weight when others can't brings them feelings of power.

Anorexics increase the possibility of health risks by overdoing it. Exercising when one's body is already depleted leads to dehydration, which causes electrolyte imbalances and heart complications, as previously described. When someone is tired and weak, working out leads to injuries, most commonly sprains and fractures. Also, a starving body requires more time to heal than does a healthy body, and since anorexics feel compelled to resume exercising before they are fully well, they are often likely to sustain even more serious injuries.

People used to really hand it to me for being so disciplined. I would workout snow, sleet, rain, or shine, just like the mailman. Acquaintances would say that I must be toned—a real hard body underneath all my layers of clothes. They had no idea how weak and tired I was all the time. I really wanted to just curl up and take a nap, but I was too driven to work off the food I'd eaten that day to let myself rest. I feared that if I didn't work out no matter how weak, sick, or tired I felt I would immediately get fat.

I planned my day around my exercise. How much I could eat depended on how long and how many times a day I worked out. I fit my friends in around my exercise schedule. I remember doing an aerobics tape, hearing the phone ringing, and my friends leaving messages on the answering machine. There was no way that I was going to stop working out to talk to them. I was too busy burning those calories and making sure my stomach stayed flat.

I used to make a schedule each day with every minute of the day accounted for. Exercise was sprinkled throughout my schedule. You know, 9:00-11:30 AM I had class, from 11:30-noon I ran laps in the gym, and was back in class till 3:00. I ran all the way home to study, and filled my study breaks with sit-ups, push-ups, and running in place—but softly, so my parents couldn't hear.

Before I was anorexic, I was a star runner. I qualified for all kinds of important races and I loved to run more than anything else in the world. But the more weight I lost, the slower I ran, and pretty soon I couldn't even qualify for races anymore. My running was helping me get thinner faster, but it was also taking away the one thing that I really loved, because pretty soon I couldn't run anymore. Since I've been eating more, I'm running again, but not to lose weight. If I stay healthy I will always be able to do this thing that makes me feel so good and that I love so much.

Is anorexia nervosa related to sexual trauma?

Numerous studies have been conducted to determine the prevalence of a history of sexual abuse in eating disorders patients, and the findings have been controversial. The figures range from 7% to 74%, with most studies showing that between 20-69% of anorexics and bulimics have been abused. The data is similar in the general population, showing a 27-67% range, which has some researchers speculating that sexual abuse is not a significant cause of eating disorders, a theory with which we do not agree. The differences in these figures probably have to do with the stigma associated with reporting incest, rape, and molestation. The fact that the incidence was thought to be only 1 in 1000 during the 1960's indicates how far we have come in disclosure. (Schwartz and Cohn 1996) Whatever the actual numbers may be, anorexia functions as a loyal shield for survivors, shifting the focus from the traumatic event to an intense preoccupation with food and weight.

It is important to note, however, that not everyone who has been sexually abused develops anorexia *and* not all anorexics have been sexually abused. The connection exists only for some people, and it is specifically for them that we elaborate.

Being sexually abused, whether once or a hundred times, is a shattering experience which evokes unbearable feelings of rage, shame, humiliation, helplessness, and grief. Survivors of abuse find many ways in which to cope with their terrifying experiences and all of the overwhelming emotions that accompany them. Some dissociate during the actual experiences and repress the memories, only to have them resurface years later. Others hide from the pain by using drugs, alcohol, food or promiscuity.

One theory proposes that people who were sexually abused had no control over what happened to their bodies, and subsequently develop eating disorders as a way of regaining that control. It contends, particularly for those who were forced to perform oral sex, that the very act of eating becomes a recreation of the trauma itself. Purging or refusing to eat then becomes a viable way to alleviate not only their immediate feelings of discomfort, but feelings of powerlessness, as well. Kathryn Zerbe, author of *The Body Betrayed,* describes this in terms of a patient:

> Her abhorrence of fellatio later manifested itself in the concrete symptom of her purging. It was nearly impossible for her to ingest any food without vomiting afterward as a way of controlling what had previously been beyond her control. Moreover, she associated any aspect of her body, including her mouth, with sex and as therefore abhorrent. Years of overstimulation were manifested in her eating disorder whereby consuming a meal repeated the trauma (p. 204).

In their chapter in the book *Sexual Abuse and Eating Disorders*, Ann Kearney-Cooke and Ruth Striegel-Moore further discuss the issue of control:

> For the eating-disordered client, regaining the safety that was lost during the abuse becomes associated with being able to restrict "bad" foods and taking in only "good" foods. Moreover, reestablishing control is associated with needing no one, with isolating oneself on an "anorexic island," with becoming a self-contained system in which one will never feel vulnerable to the betrayal of others. The need to be "perfect" to cover up the "badness," "dirtiness," "ugliness," of abuse becomes associated with being in complete control over one's appearance (e.g., not a hair is out of place), over one's needs and feelings (e.g., never feeling hunger for food, human contact, or sexuality), and over one's relationships with others (e.g., never being disappointed again) (Kearney-Cooke 1996, p. 158).

For many survivors, anorexia can also serve as a way to make their bodies less desirable to potential perpetrators. In one sense, mature adolescents deny their sexuality by returning to a prepubescent state, and in fact amenorrhea is one of the criteria for diagnosing anorexia. Another interpretation is that the individual tries to become so thin that she essentially disappears, thereby hiding not only her body, but also the shame or "badness" of her being. In this slow suicide, she feels safe.

Whatever the link—control, fear, coping strategies, or a combination of these and others—healing from sexual abuse requires compassion, caring, and tenderness from the individual as well as her caregivers. Survivors must gradually open up and talk about their experiences and feelings. When trauma is coupled with an eating disorder, the healing process becomes even more complex, but is manageable with proper pacing. Recovery is a journey that allows the participant to reclaim lost pieces of the self. With courage, endurance, and gentleness, she can rebuild what was deeply wounded or destroyed. Eileen T. Bills describes how childhood incest led to her anorexia in a chapter of the book, *Full Lives:*

Puberty brought the issues surrounding my abuse to full force. I didn't want to grow up and be a sexual human being. There was too much terror associated with that idea. A developing body, sexuality, guilt, shame, powerlessness, and being out of control were all one and the same thing . . . and I wanted none of it.

Puberty was just too painful an experience to allow to proceed. (In retrospect, I am amazed at how powerful the psyche is. I stopped menstruating even before any weight loss!) I was emotionally still eight years old. There was no hope of integrating the sexual aspects of my maturing body into me as a whole person, because I wasn't one.

I can see clearly today the choice I made back then. My body, my femininity, and my sexuality became the enemy because, if it hadn't been for these, those vile sexual acts wouldn't have occurred. I wouldn't have been prey to others who used my body—used *me*—to gratify their own selfish needs . . . I truly believed that I was . . . becoming pure by feeling the gnawing tightness in my stomach from not eating or from making special additions to my exercise routine (Hall 1993, pp. 62-65).

Monika's story, which follows in Chapter 2, is another example of the relationship between sexual abuse and anorexia. Here are comments from a few other women:

As long as I was obsessed with continually counting calories, weighing myself, working out, and striving to lose weight (and doing that successfully), I never had to deal with being sexually abused. I was too caught up thinking about food to pay any attention to how scared, dirty, and hurt I felt inside.

Being too thin distracted people from knowing me and all the secrets I carried inside from having been molested. I thought that was good because I didn't want anyone to know those things.

I am an incest survivor. I think anorexia helped me survive by keeping me unaware of my feelings connected to it.

What special issues are faced by males with anorexia nervosa?

Although an estimated 10% of anorexics are male, most clinicians see few, if any, men in their practices. Sexual orientation and certain occupations are among factors that apparently increase the risk of eating disorders in men. Statistically, homosexual, bisexual, and asexual men are shown to be higher risk groups. Men with appearance-oriented jobs such as modeling or acting and those employed in traditionally female occupations, such as nursing and food preparation, also seem to develop anorexia at a higher rate than the general male population. (Yager 1998) Most at risk are men engaged in sports which require them to "make weight," such as wrestling, crew, and gymnastics. However, despite these generalizations, males of all ages, from all backgrounds, develop eating disorders.

Men and boys develop anorexia for many of the same reasons that women do and they experience similar behaviors and feelings. Since eating disorders have been primarily considered to be a "women's disorder," the shame and guilt experienced by men may be even more pronounced and further contribute to what may already be a low sense of self-esteem. While societal pressure around thinness allows many people to "understand" a woman's anorexia, a similar compassion for men has been missing, which may be the foremost reason why clinicians have historically seen so few in treatment.

When men do enter treatment in a particular program or group, they are likely to find themselves the only male. An all male support group is rare. While some men say that they greatly appreciated the sensitivity of their female group members, others only feel even more isolated in their struggle to get well.

Also, there is not much information available for and about men with eating disorders. Although bookshelves abound with books on eating disorders and feminism, mother/father roles, and cultural pressures on women, there are fewer than a handful of books specifically focused on males and food problems. Further, education and prevention efforts have been primarily targeted at young women, when young men are equally susceptible to cultural stereotypes, often resorting to desperate means to change their bodies such as abuse of steroids and growth hormones.

Here are insights from two men:

Anorexia, once you get into the behaviors and the underlying issues, is pretty much the same whether you are male or female. I never tried to find an all-male support group or treatment center. I never felt that would be necessary. I found the women I was in treatment with to be very helpful. They always tried to understand me, and I think they did.

Sometimes it is harder to get people to understand that you are worried about your weight and that yes, you are a man. It doesn't seem to be the sort of thing you can just say to people and expect them to be empathic. Where a woman can say to someone "I am anorexic," and have people acknowledge the severity of her situation, a guy can say the same thing and people just sort of stare back with this question mark in their eyes.

How does anorexia nervosa affect relationships?

Anorexia is an isolating disorder in many ways. So much attention is devoted to food issues that there is little time left for relationships. Even when anorexics do find a way to be with family and friends, the illness stands between them. Discussions which focus on the genuine concerns about the anorexic's weight, eating, and exercise, in the hope that she will change, just add pressure. She sees fat, they see thin. She wants control, they want to take that from her.

It would seem natural, then, that the solution would be to simply stop focusing on the anorexia, allowing the relationships to deepen. Not so. The disorder itself clouds emotions and connections. Asked what they like or don't like, or how they feel, individuals struggling with anorexia are at a loss, distanced from their own answers to these questions. Their lives revolve so completely around anorexia that they have lost the most important connection of all—the one to their own selves—and along with that lost connection go thoughts and feelings about most other life issues. As long as anorexia is their best friend, they remain separated from both themselves and others.

This problem is compounded by the many celebrations and social gatherings which, in our culture as in others, center around food. An anorexic is easily overwhelmed in all of these situations which range from family meals and dorm study breaks to sports banquets, wedding receptions, and graduation buffets. In these scenarios, she finds herself fretting over how to avoid eating without drawing attention to herself and the well-meaning conversations that are sure to follow. If the pressure is too great and she simply cannot avoid eating, the remainder of the gathering is spent frantically trying to figure out how to compensate for what she did eat. Celebrations feel anything but celebratory for an anorexic, and the accompanying fears sadly take precedence over her relationships, isolating her in a secluded and lonely world.

An important step in recovery is venturing out of the rigid patterns of anorexic life and reconnecting with loved ones. As the grip of anorexia lessens, relationships become possible, as Jean Rubel, founder of one of the earliest non-profit associations in this field, Anorexia Nervosa and Related Eating Disorders, explains:

> I've finally learned to create and sustain both intimate and casual friendships, something I thought impossible when I was younger and died a thousand deaths every day from shyness. I've learned how to take the initiative, to reach out to people instead of waiting for them to notice me and take the first step. . . I've also learned to be assertive in my friendships—not selfish and demanding, but respectful of my needs as well as the other person's. If I want something, I ask for it. I don't expect

other people to read my mind or anticipate my needs. Asking for what I need was hard at first. I used to say that I'd rather be lonely than ask for quality time or a hug from someone. I felt terribly vulnerable admitting that I was not totally self-sufficient. The time came, though, when I realized that if I waited for other people to notice I needed something, I would wait a long—and awfully lonely—time (Rubel 1993, p. 47).

Here's what other anorexic women wrote about their relationships and how they changed with recovery:

The very nature of an eating disorder prevents the development of relationships. How could I have a relationship with someone based on honesty and truth if I was constantly lying about how much I ate, didn't eat, exercised, purged, etc.

Anorexia and the problems associated with it caused me to withdraw from most people. I didn't date, had few friends, and thought my family didn't care. I was afraid to go out of the house and face the world.

The sad thing is, I didn't even realize I was pushing people away. My disease blinded me. Especially when my loved ones told me I had a problem, I blocked them out even more, because hearing them drove me crazy.

My food problem destroyed the relationship between my boyfriend and me. He hated to see me slowly killing myself.

My relationships have improved dramatically in recovery. I am more open and honest, able to express my thoughts and feelings. My relationships are based on people liking me for who I am, not on what I do or how thin I can be.

Do people recover?

Absolutely! This book and many others on this topic would not exist if this were not true. Do all anorexics recover? No. Studies indicate that probably only one-third of the anorexic population fully recover, while another third reach a level of maintenance, and the remaining third continue to be chronically ill or die—many of whom never seek treatment (Zerbe, p. 250). Perhaps the more important question for readers of this book is, "Can I recover?" and the answer is a qualified yes. Clearly, those who are sincere in their desire to get better, and who are willing to work hard, have an excellent chance of completely overcoming anorexia or at least improving their current situation. Without question, anorexia is a difficult illness to treat, which is why it is so important to work with a therapist who has success and expertise in treating eating disorders.

It is important to understand that there are different ideas as to what constitutes recovery. Some people believe that recovery is an ongoing process, and that individuals with eating disorders continue to gain more perspective and perhaps maintain periods of being asymptomatic throughout their lives. Those who adhere to this "recovering" model believe that it is necessary to remain alert and aware of the fact that their eating disorder, or perhaps some other compulsive behavior, could return during periods of stress. While they firmly assert that while their eating disorder may no longer impede their ability to live life fully, they also believe that it will always be a part of them. The "recovering" or "in recovery" model, which is popular in 12-step and addictions groups, is described as it pertains to eating disorders by Caroline Adams Miller, who wrote:

While I believe that it is entirely possible to overcome an eating disorder and create "normal," guilt-free eating patterns, I also think that it is very hard for an addictive person to avoid switching to another mood-altering obsession, whether it be spirituality, sex, shopping, caffeine, alcohol, drugs, or exercising. These are the deep-seated roots that led me to abuse food in the first place, and because I'll always be the same type of personality, I'll always be in a recovering state of mind, open to new issues, new possibilities, new growth (1993, p. 148).

This particular model of recovery has many different benefits to offer those who adhere to it. For people who occasionally relapse, the "recovering" model can offer satisfying alternative explanations for the slip, preventing them from berating themselves for not being strong or committed enough. This model also offers food plans and parameters for eating which can be particularly helpful in the early stages of recovery, when eating in a healthy way can actually feel like a loss of control. Sometimes referred to as the "abstinence" approach in drug and alcohol programs, recovering anorexics are encouraged to abstain from foods or situations which might trigger their restricting behavior.

The "recovered" model, on the other hand, contends that people can become completely free from anorexia. They are able to eat a wide variety of foods, including those that they once vehemently refused to touch, without worrying about starving, purging, calorie counting, or their weight. Although much of the same work must be done no matter what the approach to recovery, this model contends that for some people, the negative thoughts and self-destructive behaviors related to the eating disorder can be completely worked through and become a part of the past.

Although both of us, Lindsey and Monika, consider ourselves to be fully "recovered," we respect both models of recovery and recognize that what works for one person does not necessarily work for another. Choose whichever approach feels right to you at your particular stage of healing, and realize that this choice is not binding. Recovery is a learning process and every victory will become an active and ongoing part of your life, no matter how the battle has been fought.

I think each person's recovery is unique and that everyone's definition of recovery is different. Personally, I will probably always be somewhat aware of my eating and weight; but, each year, the obsession lessens.

I DO believe recovery is possible. It is a day-to-day process and sometimes minute-to-minute. It is hard work, but really worth it. My life has gotten so much better.

Recovery is possible. To think otherwise is depressing, discouraging, and self-defeating. Because I believe in full recovery, it is proving true for me. I am so grateful.

There is nothing to gain by telling a starver that they are powerless. They need to learn that they have the healing power within. An eating disorder is just a symptom that something is seriously wrong in their lives. In fact, it is an invitation to grow, emotionally and spiritually. Every crisis is an opportunity. Instead of telling themselves they are powerless, they need to affirm that they are able to change and heal their lives. They may not believe it at first, but if they continue to affirm this, they will come to believe, and begin to live their authentic life.

How long does it take to get better?

There is no one answer to this question. A correlation has been found between the duration of the anorexia and the length of time it will likely take to recover; and, young patients usually progress more quickly and have a higher success rate than those who have suffered for many years. However, even those who have been chronically restricting for 20 years or more can—and do—end their obsession with thinness. Also, studies indicate that the lower the body weight at the beginning of treatment, the poorer the prognosis. Researchers who conducted a 12-year follow-up investigation showed that anorexics who started treatment at a "good" or "intermediate" anorexic weight fared better than those who were more acutely thin—at 60% or less of expected normal weight (Yager 1997a).

In the beginning stages, the tendency is to believe that recovery means achieving and maintaining a certain weight. However, as recovery unfolds, the attention shifts inward to explore the origins, onset, and progression of the eating disorder, which in turn leads to a deeper and more meaningful understanding of one's self and one's place in the world. The path of recovery is inescapably sprinkled with frustrating setbacks and plateaus, that at times may cause you to wonder if you are moving forward. However, these times are actually tremendous opportunities to learn.

No one can put a time frame on recovery. In Paul Hamburg's chapter "How Long is Long-Term Therapy for Anorexia Nervosa?" in the book, *Treating Eating Disorders,* the psychiatrist describes a six-year therapeutic relationship with a woman who had been anorexic for 17 years at the beginning of treatment. He writes:

Ms. Q's story remains unfinished, her future uncertain. Our work in therapy is far from over. What is clear is how different a person she is now than she was six years ago. From the extreme impoverishment of her anorexic world—dependent, alone, brittle, and harsh—a more complex person has emerged. She is now capable of wanting something in the world and of struggling to attain it. She is willing to overcome adversity and face loss. To sit with her now is to be in the company of another person. . .

From my labors as Ms. Q's therapist, I have learned something of inestimable value. In this current climate of therapeutic nihilism, we must remember that change is possible even when it seems least so. We cannot afford to discard individual lives because the road is so difficult and long. This work requires forbearance, extensive outside support, some inventiveness, and theoretical flexibility. We would do well to ponder what Ms. Q can teach us about the value of psychotherapy, of persistence, and of refusing to give up. (Hamburg 1996, pp. 98-99)

As we described in the previous question, recovery is a process, not an event. It is unique to each person, but in every case demands commitment, determination, and willingness. It means exploring new behaviors, developing new ways of thinking, and sitting with some inevitable emotional and sometimes physical discomfort. It requires hard work and a great deal of risk taking—not just in terms of food and weight. Recovery obliges you to open up, to discover and share parts of yourself, and to connect with the people in your life. It is a dynamic, constantly-evolving process with perspectives that continually shift.

When I think about my journey of leaving anorexia behind, I am reminded of Dorothy who had the power and tools necessary to leave OZ with her all the time. It took me several years of gradual progress to realize that I had some pretty powerful tools of my own.

Can medication help in recovery?

The role of medication in the treatment of anorexia is not conclusive. Although studies have been conducted since the late 50's, there has been no evidence of any drug having a strongly positive or direct effect. Antipsychotic medications, antidepressants, anxiolytics, and appetite-enhancing agents have all been investigated with limited outcomes (Walsh 1995, p. 313-315; Garfinkel and Walsh 1997, p. 375-377).

In the 1960's, the antipsychotic drug, chlorpromazine, was used to promote weight gain. Sometimes it was combined with insulin and bed rest, which resulted in discouraging, adverse side-effects. Cyproheptadine, an antihistamine and antiserotonergic agent that is often used to treat allergies was considered in the 70's and 80's for weight gain as well, but its benefits were minor. Likewise, benzodiazepine or lorazepam, which are taken by people with anxiety disorders, have been used during early stages of refeeding with the proviso that such usage should be strictly time-limited. More recently, dexamethasone, which affects hormone secretion, has also been studied for stimulating appetite (Yager 1997b).

Most investigators have concluded that anorexics do indeed have ample appetites but are terrified of giving in to their desires to eat. Because of their intense fear of losing control around food, many relapse after leaving inpatient settings, where appetite-enhancement methods were used. For this reason, weight restoration is often encouraged through psychotherapeutic means rather than by increasing the appetite with drugs.

For depressed anorexics, or those who also suffer from obsessive-compulsive disorder, antidepressants are sometimes used to alleviate the depression and reduce the obsessive state. The most commonly-prescribed antidepressant is fluoxetine, which is also known as Prozac®. The idea is that by feeling more hopeful and less lethargic, the patient is then able to focus and work on their eating disorder. But because depression can be a side effect of starvation, many doctors hesitate to prescribe medication before eating has been normalized, at which point many patients improve dramatically. However, when depression persists despite normal eating, antidepressants may be appropriate. In the mid-90's, Prozac received FDA approval for treating bulimia, and it has been shown to be helpful for anorexics who also binge and purge. However, antidepressants have not proven to be effective during the acute treatment phase of anorexia nervosa.

The discomfort caused by delayed gastric emptying, early satiety, and bloating, common with anorexia, can be addressed with prokinetic agents, which are usually administered intravenously. Cisapride is occasionally used to improve these symptoms and can lead to slight weight gain. However, as stressed earlier in the discussion of appetite enhancers, the benefits are limited and questionable.

The use of vitamin and mineral supplements are also considered for some anorexics. Zinc deficiency may affect loss of appetite and changes in taste, and zinc supplementation has been found to have a slight impact on some patients. Likewise, multiple vitamins may be marginally helpful.

In summary, there is no magic pill to cure anorexia. Medication should primarily be considered when other psychological disorders coexist with anorexia, including major depressive disorders, anxiety disorders, personality disorders, obsessive-compulsive disorder, and schizophrenia. Decisions about pharmacological approaches must be made in cooperation with a medical doctor, and unquestionably, the best results occur when drugs are used as an adjunct to psychotherapy and other recovery approaches. The experiences of the following voices echo these opinions:

I was really depressed. Just sad and hopeless all the time. I went on an antidepressant and it helps me function a lot better. I still have bad days, but I don't have as many now.

I've been on every medication under the sun, and none of them helped me at all. Usually I just suffered from their side effects. But I have been learning new skills and new ways of coping and treating myself. For those who don't feel better with medication, there is still a lot of hope out there!

I had a lot of trouble with anxiety. My doctor prescribed buspar and that has made a pretty big difference for me.

Will I need professional help?

Anyone with anorexia should seriously consider getting professional help for many reasons. First, professionals are just that— trained to listen, give feedback, encourage, challenge, and provide ways of coping with life other than through an eating disorder. Also, eating disorders are isolating illnesses and entering into a trusting relationship with a professional is a major step forward.

Certainly there are medical and nutritional considerations to address as well, depending on the severity of the illness. Consider consulting a treatment "team" of specialists who have experience treating eating disorders, each of whom will have a unique contribution to offer.

Anorexia can be very dangerous, and for this reason a medical doctor is an important element of treatment. Whether or not you are ready to begin the healing process, an M.D. can still monitor your physical health and insure that you are medically safe, as well as prescribe and monitor drug therapy when appropriate.

Individual therapy with a professional such as a psychotherapist, psychiatrist, marriage and family counselor, or social worker is a way to explore all of the difficult issues that led to and perpetuate your eating disorder. It provides a nurturing environment where you can learn about who you are, how you feel, what you need, and how to meet those needs in healthy ways. For many people it is the first place that they have found to express themselves and really be heard.

Family therapy, which can be extremely helpful for individuals with anorexia, is based on the idea that an eating disorder is a symptom of problems within the family system as a whole. While a family might not be the cause of an eating disorder, it might have contributed to the development or maintenance of the problem. Family therapy is a safe place where the function of the eating disorder within the family can be explored, communication skills can be learned or improved, and relationships can begin to heal and strengthen. When each member enters family therapy with an open mind and a firm commitment to honestly face and work through any and all problem areas that may arise, the experience is usually beneficial for everyone involved.

Group therapy allows for sharing thoughts, feelings, and fears with others who understand your experience. Led by a professional therapist who helps maintain the focus of the group, it is a place where members can discuss anything from food behaviors and ways to change them to the underlying issues. Group members can offer unique encouragement, support, and empathy to one another, which greatly enhances the recovery process.

Nutritionists and dieticians can help you normalize your eating by developing a plan that is both tolerable and acceptable to you. They can educate you about food and how it works in your body, dispelling myths such as the idea of "good" and "bad" foods.

The roles of each of these professionals, as well as the benefits of working with them, is discussed in Chapter 4: Get Support.

My nutritionist has been wonderful to me. She is helping me to add new foods to my diet at a reasonable pace. It's nice to have someone to talk to just about food fears who won't make you feel bad by telling you that you're being irrational. Learning about nutrition and my body's needs from her helps me to deal with my anxiety around eating foods that feel risky to me.

My therapist has been the most important person in my recovery. Talking with her about how I feel and what I think, and receiving empathy in return, have been the most healing aspects for me. It has taken a long time to really trust her and be able to share my innermost me. . . but it has been invaluable.

Group therapy has helped me the most. I can say whatever it is that I really feel and look back at other group members and see that they understand exactly how I feel. We work together to solve, and find alternative ways to cope with, the problems in our lives.

I work with a doctor, dietician, and psychologist. I learn different things from each one of them, and they have all been important and helpful to me in my recovery. I know I am making progress faster because I am working with them.

When is hospitalization necessary?

Obviously, an acute condition such as cardiac arrhythmia or organ failure warrants an immediate call to "911" or trip to the emergency room of the nearest hospital. However, hospitalization can also be necessary in non-emergency situations, where electrolytes have fallen to dangerously low levels or severe malnutrition becomes life-threatening.

In instances when the body desperately needs replenishment and the anorexic is unable (for whatever reason) to eat or drink, tube feeding might be considered. Tube feeding, or nasogastric feeding, is a process by which nutrition is supplied to the body most often through a tube inserted through the nose into the stomach. In chronic cases, the feedings are sometimes given through a tube which enters the stomach directly through an incision in the abdomen. This invasive procedure is used only in extreme cases to provide temporary nourishment. Doctors may also opt to provide liquids and nutrition intravenously. In either situation, the results are short-lived, necessary to keep the individual alive, but not effective in changing the anorexic mind-set and behavior.

Some hospitals provide intensive, inpatient, eating disorders programs which provide therapy and support as well as medical management. When the anorexia worsens in spite of individual therapy or other interventions, these programs can be just the push that a person needs to get unstuck. In addition to inpatient settings, many hospitals or other treatment facilities offer outpatient, day-hospital, residential treatment, and various support groups.

I had to be hospitalized for heart problems that I developed as a result of my anorexia. It was terrifying. I wasn't happy with my life or myself, but I wasn't ready to die because of that.

I checked myself into an eating disorders program. I wasn't about to die, but I think I was headed there. Honestly, I didn't go in because I was worried about my physical health, I went because I just couldn't live that way anymore. I was so miserable thinking about food all the time, constantly weighing myself, I forgot what fun was.

I went into the hospital because my weight was so low. I had to be fed with a tube. I never thought it would get to that point, but it did.

Going inpatient was one of the most important steps in my recovery. I kept reminding myself that I was there to begin to heal. That's really what it was, too—the beginning. The issues I identified there are issues I now work on in therapy. The coping skills I learned there are skills I now use every day.

What if I don't always want to get better?

Feelings of ambivalence are normal in the course of recovery. Anorexia is a paradox, because while it is slowly killing you, it is also serving you in some way. It is natural to fear the uncertainty of what life would be like without it. Don't expect to feel 100% committed all the time, but know with certainty that your life will be infinitely better once you are well.

Unfortunately, the solution is not as simple as just finding something healthy to substitute, because there really is no single outlet that will do all of the things that anorexia manages to do for you. Clearly, switching addictions is not a healthy alternative, although it is not unusual for people with eating disorders to become cross-addicted to alcohol or drugs, or visa versa. Of course, acquiring new positive behaviors and perspectives requires both time and effort, and it takes ongoing practice to feel comfortable with them. The temptation may be to turn back to the eating disorder, which still feels comfortable and familiar, but that is the challenge of recovery, and completely normal.

When relapses occur, try to avoid thinking of them as "failures." Instead, view them as opportunities for learning what works for you and what does not. Pain may lie beneath your eating disorder, and it takes courage and endurance to discover how to cope with this pain.

Staying focused in recovery can be hard. Anorexia was my life, anorexia was me. As I began to get better, I started feeling difficult emotions that I didn't know how to cope with. It was almost always those overwhelming feelings that would send me spinning back into my anorexia. It took me a while to figure out that even the overwhelming feelings pass.

For me it turned out to be a matter of finding good support. That took a while, and there were a lot of slips and fumbling around while I was doing that, but I did finally succeed. If I can, anybody can.

Recovery is hard and scary. Every now and then, I had to make myself do things that I didn't really want to do, but in the end, it all paid off.

CHAPTER **2**

Searching for Safety
Monika's Story

Introduction

Sometimes, as I glance back to see all that has transpired in my life, I feel nearly a hundred years old. Surely someone who has lived through so much could not have just turned thirty! I look back with sadness and pride. The sadness comes from the pain that prevailed throughout much of my life; the pride from knowing that I am doing more with that pain than just surviving it.

While it is true that I have a lengthy history of severe emotional, physical, and sexual abuse, the primary focus of this chapter will be on the portion of my life that was spent struggling with an eating disorder. This then, is mostly a description of the friend that helped me to survive, the foe that I eventually came to conquer, and the teacher that prodded me to seek wisdom and meaning—anorexia.

The Beginning

As far back as I can remember, life was about meeting challenges—and there were many to meet. The household I grew up in was filled with emotional abuse, particularly after my parents' separation when I was five. Daily life overflowed with complicated mind games and rigid, bizarre rules too complicated to capture in words. I was subjected to an inordinate amount of unspeakable sexual and physical abuse at the hands of several relatives who lived nearby. The abuse happened daily, often multiple times a day. It began at an early age and lasted until I became an adult. Although I tried several times to get someone to intervene on my behalf, I was met with little success. Abuse was something I was forced to learn to live with.

On the whole, my childhood was one that was characterized primarily by sadness, loneliness, and fear. I felt unloved, unappreciated, and worthless. I had the sense that there was something terribly wrong with me, and although I never knew exactly what it was, I was certain that it was responsible for the terrible way people treated me. I tried hard to compensate for the presence of that thing by going out of my way in attempt to please people. Every night I went to bed begging God to make me a good person. I reasoned that if I could become good, people would treat me better.

How I survived those days has never been a mystery to me. Books, writing, and school were my salvation. I immersed myself in stories about girls my own age. I could get so engrossed in the books I was reading that I'd forget about what was being done to my body and mind. I could forget about the names I'd been called; I could ignore the pain between my legs and the bruises I became so good at hiding. While I was reading, my world simply did not exist.

Writing my own stories worked much the same way. I spent hours creating happy girls with loving families and caring friends. I would pretend to be that girl who laughed and played.

School was similar. Learning kept me busy, and my classmates kept me company. School was the only place where I got to talk to or play with kids my own age. In fact, it was the only safe play I ever knew. While I was there, I smiled and acted "normal," pretending to be someone else. I kept all of the secrets I was supposed to keep, and no one had any idea that my life was anything less than ideal.

I took pride in my school work and thrived on the feedback I received. My high school teachers told me that I was a talented student with enormous potential. The work I did for the community and school as a student council officer filled me with pride and a sense of purpose. I enjoyed a job as a waitress. Both at school and work, I was reputed to be a vivacious girl with a great sense of humor. Making people laugh kept me going. A grueling schedule of classes, extracurricular activities, and work took the focus off of my painful circumstances and helped me remain optimistic until I could leave for college.

College and eighteen. The magic place, the magic number. I'd been waiting to turn eighteen so I could leave home. I wasn't bitter, just anxious. As far as I was concerned, I was going some place, and the sooner I got there the better. From the time I was very small, I was convinced that college and law school were my tickets to a better life.

Out On My Own

College was my new beginning, I told myself with a smile. I could be anybody that I wanted to be. I made new friends, participated in new classes, and immersed myself in campus activities. In a matter of weeks I was elected to secretary of my class and vice president of the Student Union. Overall, I was excited about my prospects. I had received enough scholarship money to be able take the first semester off work, and I fully intended to enjoy college life. But the first semester passed quickly and along with it my optimism. I didn't have to study much to get excellent grades, and the pervasive, high level of apathy on campus drained my enthusiasm. Despite being academically uninspired and socially disappointed, I vowed to make the best of it until I could transfer to Wellesley the following year.

Second semester was a prominent time marker. I was busier than ever, having added my first serious relationship to my schedule. But more notable—it was the semester I gained weight. I had always had the kind of metabolism that allowed me to eat anything without a thought. I was accustomed to people telling me that I was thin, so I didn't mind when I put on five pounds during the first semester. After I started taking birth control pills, however, I put on ten more pounds and suddenly my clothes were too tight. I felt bloated, fat, self-conscious, and uncomfortable. Where five pounds had been okay, 15 was completely unacceptable; I wanted my old body back.

Immediately I vowed to lose weight, and headed off to the bookstore in search of diet books that would tell me how to do it. Amidst those pages I learned about calorie counting, and went on to research dieting in books, pamphlets, magazines. I spent hours gazing at magazine pictures of the models' flat stomachs, determined that mine would look that way.

I read that if you ate 1200 calories a day you could lose between one and two pounds a week, far too long to wait in my impatient opinion. My plan was simple: I would eat between 300-600 calories a day. I also began running, doing sit-ups, karate, and aerobics in order to speed my weight loss. It wasn't long before I went home to find the scale reading 113 pounds, exactly one pound below my pre-college weight. When I saw the number, my first thought was, "That's safe." My relief was fleeting, however, and an obsessive rigidity quickly took its place. I had spent too many miserable hours fretting about my unexpected weight gain and trying to get rid of it, and I never wanted to repeat that process again. I resolved to never let the scale budge even one ounce above the number 113.

Just to be safe, I calculated the caloric intake for a shorter, more sedentary person than myself, and then proceeded to keep meticulous track of everything I put in my mouth—including gum, cough drops, and antacids. That was also when I became a *bona fide* slave to the scale. The scale was my first stop in the morning, right after the bathroom. If I liked the number, I would be in a fairly good mood. If I didn't like the number, I would vow to be more vigilant and feel angry and miserable most of that day. I checked my weight several times throughout the day and always before going to bed—again—just to be safe. It was the only way to ensure that my weight would never again take me by surprise.

My rigidity progressed, as I constantly came up with new rules. I did not allow myself to eat in the dining hall, because there was no way to be certain how many calories existed in the food. Soon I stopped eating breakfast entirely, and lunch diminished to one slice of tomato sprinkled with salt and pepper on diet toast. My list of off-limits foods grew daily. I had a terrible penchant for sweets, but chewing gum managed to quell most of my cravings—most, but not all. There was always some point in the week when I would come face to face with cookies, chocolate, or some other forbidden food. Sometimes I'd give in and eat a little, which would make me feel terribly guilty. I was also careful to make up for each of my transgressions by either cutting more food out of my dwindling diet or by adding more exercise to my already too-strict regime.

Each year of college was distinct for something that I was doing to either lose or maintain my weight. Sophomore year was the year I took laxatives, but that didn't last long because it caused more discomfort than it was worth. Junior year was the year I discovered throwing-up, which seemed like the perfect solution to eating past my limit. I figured that if I ate a cookie or two, I could simply vomit afterwards. Once I realized that I couldn't always purge successfully, however, I returned to my more reliable extra workouts and two-day fasts. Senior year was more eclectic: I did a little of everything. I never missed my daily five-mile run and did hundreds of sit-ups and calisthenics in my room. I continued to religiously keep track of everything that passed my lips, while occasionally taking laxatives, and making myself throw up.

I thought that going to college would be the solution to my problems at home, but in truth, it changed nothing. In addition to the abuse from family members when I went home on vacations, I also began having serious problems with my boyfriend. His heavy drinking made him angry and controlling. Furthermore, although transferring to Wellesley College was a sound academic choice, I had difficulty making friends there. Between my work schedule, classes, domineering boyfriend, and weight-loss regime, I didn't have time left to cultivate and nurture friendships. I had waited my whole life for college to free me, and I was anything but free. My only alternative was to wait for law school.

If the only way to go is up, why am I sinking?

Ironically, life in law school was nothing like I'd imagined. I kept up with the work and my waitressing job, but I had no time for friends or meaningful activities. My boyfriend was more violently abusive than ever, and the emotional torment from my family increased. The boundaries and limits I arduously tried to set were ignored, and the message that I was unimportant and worthless echoed loud and clear. I was about as miserable as one could get. In typical fashion, I figured it was just a matter of hanging in there for the three years until I graduated—then I would finally have my JD and a better life.

Also in characteristic style, I decided that I needed to lose a little more weight. I feared that my first year of law school would be a replay of my first year in college. So, just to be safe, I devised a few new rules: I had to run wherever I went, I had to take the longest route to get there, and I could never use an elevator. I stuck to a strict, explicit schedule, waking each morning at dawn to head straight out to run for no less than one hour. I spent class time listening, taking notes, briefing cases and answering questions if I was called on, while simultaneously calculating my caloric intake and expenditure in the margins of my notebooks.

In the evening, I followed a 15-minute, video aerobics routine, which I would do precisely ten times in a row—and it had to be exactly ten times. Once I even awoke at 3 a.m. panic stricken because I couldn't remember how many times I had done the video that day. It might have been nine times, it might have been ten. But because I couldn't say for sure, I got out of bed and worked out one more time just to be safe.

During that time, my food intake was limited to snacking on a few pieces of hard candy or carrot sticks during the day and nonfat sugar-free yogurt or a slice of diet bread for a meal. Sometimes I treated myself with a diet soda and one miniature Reeses peanut butter cup, but if I ate anything else, I threw it up.

By the time I reached the low 80 pound range, I was constantly weak and tired, but I didn't care. I had difficulty concentrating and would have to read the same page multiple times. I pushed myself to continue my exercise regime despite the fact that I was starting to feel sick. My stomach burned horribly, and I was throwing up blood. An endoscopy revealed tears in my esophagus and severe gastritis, for which I was given a Zantac prescription. The only person who ever thought to question me about an eating disorder was an internist in an emergency room. Although his question evoked panic, I calmly looked him in the eye and denied having any problems with food.

Continually lowering my goal weight was not logical, and I knew that. None of my food or weight goals made sense, but still I could not relinquish them. Every day I promised myself that I would eat or that I wouldn't throw up, and every day I broke that promise. My obsession with food and weight seemed to have sneaked up on me and taken over my life. Somewhere in the maze of my rigid routines and beliefs about food and weight, all of my other goals and interests had vanished. I was in trouble and I knew it. I resolved to see a therapist.

I went through the initial interview answering all of the questions with great hesitation. I had learned early on that telling my secrets only brought trouble, and I was wary. I didn't like that particular therapist, but that turned out to be irrelevant. She required that I see a medical doctor before she would work with me, and when the doctor took one look at my weight and lab results, he insisted that I enter the hospital for tube feeding. I was shocked. I recognized that my fear of food and weight gain had reached a phobic level, but it seemed much more logical to combat that fear by eating real food in a supportive environment. My other pressing concern was that I was in the middle of final exams. I mentioned to the doctor that law school didn't seem to be a place that granted extensions, and I was worried about completing my first year. Without commenting on my academic obligations, he told me that my body had gone into something called ketosis and that I was at serious risk for a heart attack.

He continued to insist that I sign myself into the hospital. Despite his urgent tone of voice and explicit statements, I couldn't make myself believe that I was in danger. I didn't know what the word ketosis meant, and I didn't think to ask. It didn't sound all that serious to me. And while I watched his lips form the words "heart attack," I could not make myself understand that they applied to me. There was something very surreal about it. So, I told the doctor that I would go home to think about it, but if I decided to go in, it wouldn't be until my exams were completed the following week.

My mind was far more optimistic than my body. I returned home to study and work, but the weekend was rough. I wasn't able to study, and I got lost on a highway I drove nearly everyday. I passed out on the way up the stairs and again on the bathroom floor. I thought a shower would make me feel better, but the water hurt as it hit my skin. When I got out of the shower I felt dizzy and had trouble breathing. That night, for the little time that I did manage to sleep, I dreamed that I died. The following morning, I was scared enough to call the doctor and agree to hospitalization the following day.

Treatment Daze

I arrived at the hospital both apprehensive and optimistic. The admissions procedure didn't take much longer than half-an-hour. They checked my vital signs and weighed me with my back to the scale, a customary practice for eating disorder patients. Once the admission routine was complete, I was brought to my room where I sat shivering on my bed waiting for the doctor to arrive and insert the tube. Although I was certain that things would now start to turn around, I was still nervous. It wasn't long before the doctor came bounding into the room, greeting me with cheerful words of encouragement. After several painful tries, he finally got the tube inserted down the back of my throat.

Shortly after I walked into the bathroom, dragging the pump behind me, catching a brief sideways glimpse of myself in the mirror. Oddly, it wasn't the tube taped to the side of my nose that caught my eye, it was the bruises that ran all the way down my spine. They were big, black, and ugly. At first I was baffled. I wasn't sure where they had come from. Then I realized that they were from sitting in the bathtub and hard chairs at law school. There were no words to form a thought, only a sad feeling as I shook my head.

The two weeks I spent on the tube were long and uncomfortable. I developed a constant sore throat and the feeding solution felt like lead pouring into my stomach. I developed edema, and although the swelling wasn't terribly severe I had to wear special stockings to help with the discomfort. I was bored in my room, with far too much time on my hands to worry about all the calories that were gushing into my body. The nurses brought three trays of food a day. I was supposed to work up to eating at least

75% before I would be taken off the tube and allowed to enter the eating disorders program. I never reached that goal, however. With all of the tube calories I was already ingesting, I was too afraid to take more than an occasional bite.

Everyday I would have a 30 minute session with one of the therapists. I tried to talk about my anxiety which stemmed from the tube calories, and how scared I was to eat, but he wouldn't let me, telling me that discussions about food and weight were off limits. Suddenly I felt ashamed that I had those fears. He went on to tell me that all anorexics are manipulative, and that he knew I was too. He also told me that eating disorders are maladaptive coping techniques. Listening to him made me feel backed into a corner. What could I do with my anxiety if I couldn't talk about it? I managed it by continuing not to eat from the trays.

After several days of not eating, the doctor, nutritionist, and therapist all came in to push me to try harder. They encouraged me by telling me that I was a good patient because I wasn't exercising in my room. My eyebrow raised a little. Exercising in my room—hmm!—now why hadn't I thought of that? I started eating a little and made up for it by doing jumping jacks, sit ups, and portions of the aerobics tape that I'd memorized. It was difficult to exercise on the tube, and I knew that I wasn't burning a significant amount of calories, but it alleviated the monstrous level of anxiety that had consumed me from the beginning of tube feeding. Soon after I started eating, I was taken off the tube and admitted to their full-fledged eating disorders program.

The program itself was behaviorally based and consisted of a thirty minute therapy session combined with all-day groups. The rules around food were simple: I had three days to eat 100% of my daily meals, snacks and supplements or I'd be discharged. My biggest problem stemmed from the fact that while I had been on the tube I had eaten no more than the total of a couple bites of a sandwich. It had been quite a while since I had eaten solid food; and as soon as I started eating a significant amount I got sick. My body could not yet tolerate things like roast beef, chicken, and potatoes. The nurses and doctors accused me of purging, but my reaction was beyond my physical control. Still, they did not believe me.

It feels awful to tell the truth and not be believed. Their contempt was a thread that wove its way through my entire hospitalization. I was reprimanded for questioning the decisions and policies I didn't agree with or understand. They interpreted my queries as being, "hung up on control." I was stunned. I certainly never felt in control of anything, especially my anorexia. If anything, it controlled me! I was ashamed of the things that had happened to me, the way I looked, and the behaviors I couldn't stop. When I tried to explain myself, I was told that I was being manipulative and resistant to treatment.

During this admission, I mostly felt confused by the accusations and disrespect. I was unaccustomed to being abused that way by anyone outside my family. Teachers, professors, peers, coworkers, and bosses had always treated me with respect, and I was known for my honesty and good intentions. Throughout this hospitalization I had the strong instinct to leave. In my heart I knew this program wasn't right for me. But I ignored my internal guidance and listened instead to my logical mind, which told me that these were trained professionals who knew more than I did. In retrospect, I wish that my heart had prevailed, for I now know that these were not the compassionate professionals who could have helped me.

Unfortunately, I persisted in this program, believing it held the key to my recovery. I was eating more food than I had in years, but still wasn't gaining weight fast enough. More food was always added to my tray, increasing the anxiety that filled each day. I managed to ride out my fears until the day I stepped on the scale and heard the balance being moved to its next setting. That meant I weighed at least 100 pounds; I wasn't prepared for this. Overcome with panic I couldn't voice, I did the only thing I could do: purge. I felt guilty, but knew I would be publicly reprimanded and humiliated if I spoke up. So, I remained silent, worrying constantly that I would never get better.

By the end of my admission I had lost five of the pounds I'd gained, was purging regularly, and even bingeing!. The hospital staff wanted me to stay longer in order to gain more weight and work on my abuse issues. It was that last part that sent me running out the door. I was unable to talk about the abuse—I just wasn't ready—but they had pushed the issue to the point that I was having terrible nightmares. Perhaps if the therapists there had been more caring and supportive, I would have opened up to them. Instead, I left the hospital against medical advice, moved back home, and promptly lost all the weight I had gained.

Outpatient Haze

When I left, the hospital connected me to a therapist who shared their philosophy. She told me that my eating disorder was a "maladaptive coping technique" and a "distorted survival strategy that was ultimately a symptom of my disordered self." Hearing those negative statements from someone I'd only just met made me feel even worse. She could have simply said that anorexia helps people survive difficult circumstances, but it ravages the body, mind, and spirit in the process. She also could have honored the fact that I did the best I could at the time with the resources available to me, and she could have done that while encouraging me to move forward without shaming me. But she didn't. I felt uncomfortable and self-conscious in her presence, but since I had nothing to compare it to, I assumed that that was how therapy was.

This therapist primarily wanted to talk about the abuse, which was difficult. When I had told people about it before, I was physically tortured or betrayed. Telling my secrets always got me hurt, but I couldn't seem to make her understand that. She cornered me, saying that it was the only way for me to get better, and threatening that if I didn't talk about those issues she would stop working with me. Because I was under the impression that I needed her, I tried. I was detached when I talked, which she labelled as "abnormal." She also began asking me if there was anyone who could "corroborate my story," emphasizing the word "story." I was telling the absolute truth, but I had no way to prove it. My therapist didn't believe me, and what she did believe, she blamed on me.

The way the hospital clinicians had treated me, along with the way my therapist treated me, successfully eroded any remaining self-respect I had. I began to believe that I really was worthless. Never once did it occur to me to look for a new therapist. I just figured all therapists must be the same; and, because I believed I needed a therapist to heal, I stayed with the one I had.

Not returning to law school was the one good choice I did manage to make. I had been miserable there, and I desperately wanted to do something that would make me feel good. I moved in with a friend and found a wonderful job teaching social studies at a small Catholic high school. Teaching occupied my mind and gave me a sense of purpose. I was liked by the faculty and students, and I believed that I had found my niche. Despite the happiness and relief teaching provided, though, I was still caught up in the dangerous cycle of starving and purging. Regardless of my frighteningly low weight, gaining was still my greatest fear. The same rigid food rules and beliefs dominated my life, with two exceptions: I no longer exercised or weighed myself—I threw out my scale. Obsessive weighing was replaced by checking my clothes: I could easily tell how much I weighed by how they fit.

My eating, health, and weight continued to decline. Upon my therapist's persistent urging, I reentered the same eating disorders program I had been in the previous summer. Although I had despised my first admission, I still believed they could help me. By then, anorexia had become a prison from which I desperately wanted to escape.

From Darkness to a Glimmer

That second admission was a nightmare too, and I spent the next four years in and out of hospitals. I was miserable. The hospital clinicians either discounted my pain or blamed me for it. They focused instead on my intellect and how much I had to give to the world. They constantly reasoned that because I was smart enough to graduate from Wellesley, I was smart enough to stop my eating disorder. The fact that no one heard or believed me hurt. I coped by using my eating disorder and self-destructive inclinations.

After such a long time of being blamed or not believed, I started second-guessing myself and wondering if maybe I really was crazy after all. Could it be possible that it was all in my head? I began to think that I had to be really sick to think up those twisted things. I vacillated between doubting myself and my reality, to knowing with all my heart that what I said was the truth.

Finally, during one of my admissions I met a therapist whom I immediately liked. It didn't take long to know that she was the one with whom I wanted to work. She was different from anyone I'd ever met. She was gentle and patient, and although I didn't know it then, she also believed in me. The only relief I ever got from the constant soul-consuming ache was when I was in session with her. Something about her presence comforted me.

This new therapist encouraged me, but I didn't get very far. It seemed that at the end of every session I would resolve to trust her and tell her more next time. Then I'd walk out of her office, and onto the unit, where I was met by nurses who told me I was a waste of time. This obviously hurt, and I was convinced that my therapist would become so impatient with my lack of progress she'd stop working with me. This situation, coupled with my previous therapy experience, made it impossible for me to trust her. I was okay with this, however, because the only thing that mattered was that she was nice. Her kindness kept me in therapy.

Not long after meeting my new therapist, I met the man whom I would eventually marry. He, too, believed in me, but just as with my therapist, I was unable to believe him. He offered me his compassion, and only wanted to share his life with me. The problem was that I no longer wanted to live mine.

I desperately wanted to break free from my eating disorder and self-injurious behaviors, and more than anything else I wanted the constant aching to stop. I doggedly searched for answers in books, reading everything I could find on eating disorders. I tried medications, participated in therapy groups, and saw various doctors, all to no avail.

Near the end of those four years I suddenly realized something devastating. I recalled the days that I had been a talented student with many friends who treated me with respect. I remembered my optimism and how I could smile and make other people laugh. I thought about my determination, and how I used to strive to reach goals. It felt like a million years ago. What happened? Where did it go? Not only did anorexia sneak up on me and take over my life, but somewhere in just a moment's time I had made the transition from successful, respected student with a bright future to what I though was a sinking, screwed-up mental patient with no hope.

The Awakening

Ironically, the turning point came when my therapist went on a five-month maternity leave. My weight dropped to a critical point, and I knew I had to find an eating disorders program. Due to a lack of facilities, coupled with restrictions from my insurance company, I entered the same one I'd gone to years back. The program had moved to a new hospital, which made me hopeful. Something in me was changing. I was determined not only to recover, but to feel better. I recognized that the majority of my treatment had been damaging and hurtful, and I did not want that trend to continue. This time I was adamant about taking an active role in my treatment.

Most of the staff was the same, and my hope rapidly diminished. A psychologist gave me a list of conditions that I had to meet or else I would be tube-fed. He used the same old condescending tone, and once he left, I sat on my bed feeling alone and vulnerable. Just as years before, my heart was telling me to leave the program because it didn't feel right. Unlike before, this time I listened. I called my husband and said, "I know I need to be someplace, but this isn't it. Come get me, I'm signing out."

After some arduous research and digging, I managed to find a new program and entered it. This one also had a trauma track—just what I needed. It was there that I finally learned that recovery from anorexia was possible. The caring and respect that took place within its walls was miraculous, unlike anything I'd ever experienced. I was starting to feel empowered. The physician was compassionate and optimistic, willing to explain my medical situation in comprehensible terms. Groups brimmed with empathy as people shared in intimate ways. I found hope and comfort in my conversations with the other women, some of them with histories as lengthy and complicated as my own. Bound by common goals and struggles, we shared healing and strength.

One woman in particular greatly inspired me. What struck me most was that despite the humiliating things that she had been through, she treated herself with kindness. She had found her own worth and believed in herself. She shared her experiences and feelings with dignity, and I sensed that she could teach me a lot.

In Healing There is Light

I stayed in the program for nine months, driving daily over an hour just to get there. I listened, watched, and absorbed information like a sponge. I recognized my destructive patterns, and identified many of my fears. But after nine months I also realized that I was stuck. My weight reached a plateau, and I was terrified to move beyond the 100 pound mark. I knew that I had to work on my perceptions of food, weight, and myself, but I realized it needed to be done primarily on my own.

Recalling all of the behaviors I had practiced just to be safe, I understood how anorexia helped me survive. More importantly, I also understood that as long as I had anorexia, I would never be able to experience life beyond survival mode. I wanted to be free from my obsessive thoughts and rigid behaviors, and most of all I wanted to be free from the pain that filled my soul. Instinct told me that in order for that to happen, I would need to face my demons and deal with my past. Only then could I move on to find peace and fulfillment. It occurred to me that the only thing in my way was anorexia. With that realization, anorexia became the foe that I was determined to beat.

My therapist returned and I tackled my healing with her un-flagging support. The chorus of doctors and nurses disappeared, no longer able to muffle her voice. Now that she was the only person with whom I was working, I finally began to trust her belief in me.

After years of searching, I came to realize that recovery is a combination of determination, trial-and-error, journeying to self-acceptance, and practicing this with a warrior spirit. I understood that my prior treatment had been unsuccessful mainly because it felt disempowering and damaging, seeing me not as an individual but a statistic. I began to analyze what was missing in my treatment and provide it for myself.

My last admission had shown me the importance of compassion and empathy, and revealed the healing that results from loving connections. Maintaining that comfort, compassion, and understanding, however, wasn't so simple. Although my therapist had plenty to give, I didn't yet feel worthy. People in my last program had often said, "You should take better care of yourself," and "You should love yourself." But I didn't know how, simply because I hated myself about as vehemently as one could hate anything.

I thought about the women I knew who had recovered from eating disorders. What did they have in common? Suddenly I had an epiphany: they accepted who they were. They knew how to herald their successes, be patient with their flaws, and gentle with their pain.

My understanding of recovery deepened. I needed to feel worthy of compassion in order for it to work, and I had to accept who I was in order to feel worthy. I certainly had my work cut out for me! I knew in my heart that my recovery hinged on my ability to move from intense self-loathing into the realm of gentle self-love. All I had to do was plot the course.

Being a logical person, I understood that it would be a process. I began by writing about treating myself with gentleness and compassion and exploring being nonjudgmental. After writing about it, I tried it. For an entire day I refused to allow myself to label anything I thought, said, or did as good or bad. I accepted everything as simply existing. The exercise highlighted the disdain I had for myself, and I saw the great distance I had to travel before I would be able to feel consistently loving.

Part of learning to be gentle and compassionate with myself meant changing my vocabulary. I incorporated loving words into my journal entries, therapy sessions, letters to friends, and especially in my own self-talk. Whenever I had a harsh thought about myself, I would simply say, "Be gentle." I also began to visualize treating myself that way. I regularly closed my eyes and envisioned situations, while paying close attention to my internal responses. If my reaction felt judgmental or rigid, I reconstructed it to be more gentle and accepting.

In daily journal entries I wrote what I did not yet believe, to make them feel more tangible. For example, I wrote that instead of hurting myself in times of pain, I needed to allow myself to cry and be surrounded by people who cared about me. This was difficult because I wasn't sure yet that there was anyone who truly cared about me. I continually affirmed that I needed to connect with people instead of isolating out of fear of being hurt.

Through writing and therapy I explored why I didn't feel entitled to my feelings. I adopted a "say it anyway" philosophy—meaning I would say whatever I felt or thought, which helped develop my authentic voice. Anorexia's more passive-aggressive voice was on its way out.

Within the pages of my journal I explored many topics—food, trauma, feelings about myself. Because I could write I could not say, I often shared what I wrote with my therapist. This made it easier for me to initiate discussions about painful topics and seek reassurance for my new behaviors and ways of thinking.

After a good deal of writing and talking, the next logical step was to stop all of my destructive behaviors—cold turkey. Sometimes the impulses and urges were so strong I sat on my hands and witnessed the raw, edgy way I felt. I was like an addict going through withdrawal; I just had to ride it out.

I sat down with pictures of myself as a little girl. Because my self-hate was still with me, it was impossible to recognize her, and I felt compelled to make cruel comments. In order to be more objective, I pretended it was someone else. I looked at the tiny little wrists and fingers, shimmering blond hair, and big blue eyes. I closed my eyes and imagined meeting this little girl. When I imagined her talking and laughing, I felt a desire to take care of her, love her. I imagined taking her out for ice cream, my heart melting from the smile that brightened her face. I imagined watching her chase butterflies in an open field; my spirit delighting in her playfulness. I made all of the scenarios as detailed and vivid as possible, and I fell in love with this precious child.

Little by little I integrated my history into her life. Taking my most horrible memories, I pretended that they happened to her. Eventually, I came to understand that she was really *me*, and for the first time in my life the tears streaming down my face were tears of compassion. I remember that day clearly: I was sitting on my living room floor with the pictures spread out in front of me, as a soul-shattering pain filled my being.

Once gentleness for myself came, I began challenging the harmful beliefs I was holding. I became aware how I had been taught my subservience while subjected to painful manipulations. I asked and tried to answer questions like, "What is it about me that makes people treat me in hurtful ways?" and the hardest question of all, "Why?" These are questions that I have so far been unable to answer, and "Why?" continues to gnaw at my spirit.

I could not shake the feeling that there was something about me that made me a worthless person, somehow different from everyone else. I had always blamed myself for the awful things that had happened to me. I desperately wanted someone to say that it wasn't me or my fault, but I also knew that this was something I would have to discover on my own. And finally I did, accidentally, while spending time with children. Being around children taught me that every child is special and vulnerable, so greatly in need of love and protection. Soon I realized that I had been no different from any of them. More painful questions arose as I saw only too clearly what it was that my own family threw away.

The more my compassion grew, the gentler I became, the more I began to see myself as my own perpetrator. My mind and body had been through years of unspeakable abuse, and there I was subjecting them to my own destruction and self-loathing. In this way, I was like others who had hurt me before. How hard it was to look from this perspective! Because, you see, it is impossible to purposefully hurt something you love.

I diligently challenged my perspectives, asking tough questions, searching my soul, taking risks, and changing the ways I thought about myself and my world. Simultaneously, I tackled my concrete fears and rules related to food. I kept an extensive goals notebook in which I devised many exercises to challenge them. For example, each day, in order to desensitize myself from food fears, I would force myself to eat something that scared me. Then I would panic. I worried about it making me fat, about all sorts of things. I tried to figure out how I could skip dinner, purge, or use my other usual remedies to compensate. I allowed myself to panic for exactly five minutes, before I would say out loud, "WHO CARES?! IT'S JUST A CANDY BAR! SO WHAT?!?!" Then I would force myself to stop panicking by diverting my attention to something else. Sometimes it helped to recall that my recovered friends regularly ate such foods without becoming fat. Other times it helped to get out of the house. Whatever I chose, I always refused to act on my impulses to skip a meal or purge.

This particular exercise helped me expand my diet to the point where I looked like someone who had never had an eating disorder. It also helped me to be able to go anywhere and eat anything without obsessing, panicking, or driving the people I was with crazy. Most importantly, it was instrumental in diminishing my urges to purge. In fact, not too long after engaging in this practice my urges to purge disappeared entirely!

Making the weight restoration process easier and more comfortable was always of paramount importance. Staying off all scales once I had reached a safe weight meant I no longer had a number in my head to obsess about. Wearing soft, comfortable, loose clothing was also helpful. The softness felt comforting to my skin, while the looseness lessened the panic I would experience whenever my waistbands felt even the slightest bit tighter. I also forced myself to stop habitually checking the size of my stomach throughout the day. To encourage and reassure myself, I practiced copious amounts of positive self-talk, constantly affirming that my body was becoming healthy and strong. I hung affirmations all over our home, wrote them in my journal, and repeated them to myself in the car while I was driving. Changing my perception of an acceptable weight also proved to be beneficial. I began looking at normal weight women, affirming silently to myself, "That is a normal, healthy weight, and that is what I want for myself." Although I didn't believe it at first, over time I did.

Finally, with the practice of self-love and increased self-awareness came my long-awaited freedom from the prison of anorexia.

Lessons Learned

Recovering from anorexia allowed me to embark on a profound journey of healing. I have come to learn that in wounds there lies wisdom, and in healing is strength. I have come to embrace struggling as a vehicle for growth. Not only did I free myself from the prison of food and weight, but I found the perseverance and compassion necessary to tackle healing from my painful past. My journey has taught me the importance of listening to, trusting, and ultimately following my heart. It was my quest for gentleness that helped me to see that I do not deserve to be hurt by anyone—including myself. And while I will still make sacrifices for others, I no longer sacrifice myself.

In my search for the truth, I connected with a female cousin, who I had suspected experienced similar abuse. We met and found ourselves finishing each other's sentences. It was both validating and shocking to discover that my memories were correct. Sometimes I look back on my years of treatment and wonder: What if I had been believed? What if I had been offered compassion and empathy instead of accusations and blame? What if I had met my current therapist first? These are questions to which I'll never know the answers.

I have gleaned treasures from even my most difficult experiences. Because people have been quick to judge me, I am careful to give others the benefit of the doubt. I emerged from a brutal situation with a capacity to love, nurture, and care deeply about others. Knowing depths of shame, humiliation, and loneliness has given me humility, a trait that greatly enriches my life. Spending most of my life having my own feelings ignored allows me to connect with others on a meaningful, compassionate level. Regardless of the severity of the storm, I know that if I look hard enough, I will always find the rainbow.

My personal life has flourished since my recovery, and life is better than ever. Shortly after I recovered there was a period where it felt as if my husband and I had just met, and we fell in love all over again. It was a breathtaking, beautiful experience for us both. Today we find joy in planning our future, enjoying each other's company, and taking time to play. We look forward to starting our own loving family together.

My relationships with friends have also deepened. These days I have much more of myself to share. I have ambitions, goals, hopes and dreams. I experience a fulfilling peace and freedom that I never could have known while living with anorexia. I remember how to celebrate my successes and appreciate my qualities; I am patient with my flaws and gentle in times of pain. I live each day leading with my heart and following with my head.

Recovery has brought me many gifts, and today I am dedicated to helping others through their own journeys. I write, speak, and conduct workshops on recovery which emphasize the importance of following one's heart to health and healing. I am always struck when so many people approach me at the end of a lecture or workshop to tell me of their struggle, and to ask for guidance. I give from my heart and feel honored to foster their healing. My mission is to offer hope and bring light into their darkness.

I often recall the days I believed recovery was a fantasy, and am pleased to assure that it isn't—recovery is both possible and attainable. Patience and compassion, from clinicians and sufferers alike, play a fundamental role in the process, and should never be underestimated. My early experiences in treatment compel me to remind others that treatment must empower as it recognizes and builds upon the unique strength of each individual. Should treatment not feel that way, it may be time to move on to some that does. There are many empathic clinicians out there who support the challenging and rewarding journey. Recovery is a process, a struggle—one well worth the effort. I urge you to find your voice. Be gentle with your heart, and fall in love with yourself—the best is yet to be.

CHAPTER 3

Where to Start

Choose Life

The first step in recovering from anorexia is simply to *choose life*. You don't even have to know *how* in order to make this choice, but you must affirm, at a very basic level, that you want to live. Think about it: anorexia does not really allow you to live—it enables you to survive, and sometimes just barely that.

Think back to a recent important event. It could be a vacation, graduation party, wedding, or night out with friends. Did you look forward to it, or were you obsessing about food and calories? Did you laugh and have fun, or were you concentrating on ways to avoid eating? Did you converse with other people, or did you carry on an inner dialogue about your weight and worthlessness?

Can you see how anorexia seeps into all aspects of your experience? It distances you from yourself and others, preoccupies your mind, numbs your feelings, ruins your health, and diminishes the quality and meaning of almost everything that you do. What you think you are controlling is really controlling you. It may be slowly killing you.

You can do *more* than just survive in this world; you can *live* in it. If you are willing to work hard on your recovery, you can transform your life into one that feels rewarding and fulfilling. This requires being patient, present, and accepting during all stages of your progress. It also means looking at yourself objectively, and getting to know who you really are. Choosing life means believing that someday—regardless of how long it takes—you will be free.

Even if you are not completely sure that you want to begin your recovery today, *something* made you pick up this book— the possibility that things could be different, your hope for a better future, your will to live. Follow that instinct; it comes from your heart. You are the only one who can make this choice. You are the only one who can give yourself a real chance to recover. Find the courage to take this first step... be brave and choose life!

The following are quotes from individuals who discovered that their recoveries began with this one decision:

When I began to understand that anorexia is a selfish friend, I could begin to sever my ties with it. Deciding to get better meant that I had to break that friendship and lose the one thing that was always there for me.

Anorexia took up my whole life. It consumed my thoughts and dictated everything I did. I finally realized I wasn't living at all, I was just existing. I wasn't sure I deserved more than that, but I was determined to find out. Part of finding that out entailed leaving anorexia behind. I clearly remember making that decision, because it was the most important decision of my life.

Recovery was a decision for me. It was a scary decision, but when I began to understand how serious the anorexia was, it became a necessary decision.

I definitely decided to recover. To make it feel more firm, I wrote the word "anorexia" on a slip of paper, put it in a small box, and buried the box in the ground. That was the day my anorexia died. I have been devoted to living my life ever since. It was a huge struggle in the beginning, but I made a commitment to myself and stuck with it. My life has gotten much better.

Willingness and Courage

Crucial to your recovery is your willingness to do whatever it takes to get better, even if this scares you. Willingness is not the same thing as willpower. You may have tremendous willpower—most anorexics do—but it probably won't help you to fight your eating disorder. A willingness to try new things, coupled with the courage to sit through fear and discomfort are two of the most powerful, effective weapons you can have.

Recovery naturally challenges you and demands that you take risks. You need to be willing to face those challenges, to try any possibility and test it, even if you are hesitant. Be willing to endure the discomfort and anxiety that accompanies new ways of being. How else will you grow? How else will you find alternatives to the anorexia?

While it is important to experiment with new foods and different attitudes towards weight, recovery also requires that you explore the issues that led to and now maintain your eating disorder. This can be hard and uncomfortable work. In fact, as your recovery progresses, new challenges will arise seemingly out of nowhere. Remind yourself often that recovery is a process, not an event. It takes time to work through feelings, and to understand and accept your past and your present. Arming yourself with a courageous and willing attitude is not easy, but it is one of the biggest and most important steps that you can take.

During recovery I took a lot of frightening risks. Sometimes the risk was eating something I was terrified of, other times it was trusting someone with a piece of myself that I hadn't yet shared. I'm convinced that all of the risks I took were crucial to my recovery.

People give you a lot of suggestions in recovery. The trick is to keep an open mind and give everything a fair shot. Unless the suggestion sounded totally off-the-wall, I made myself try it. Sometimes I tried things more than once, because I recognized that I had only given it a half-hearted effort.

I have attempted therapy over and over again, and I'm at it for the fourth time. I moved all by myself from one state to another and I am very proud of myself. Although therapy is hard work, I now have a great support group, a good job, and I am determined to get well. Anorexia no longer serves any function in my life.

Listen to Your Inner Voice

Everyone has a quiet voice of wisdom and compassion that dwells within. This voice, which can be imagined as the voice in the heart, comes from the deepest center of being and is a source of perfect understanding and love. It offers guidance whenever we need it, but especially in recovery when we are getting to know and trust ourselves at the most profound level. Individuals with eating disorders find it particularly difficult to hear this voice because their minds are constantly racing with obsessive thoughts and critical self-talk. An important aspect of recovery, then, is learning to block out the negative voices so you can hear your loving, inner truth that serves your best interests.

If you pay attention, your critical, anorexic voice is easy to recognize because it is the loudest. No matter what the origin—parental expectations, cultural ideals, religious tenets or other source—it makes you feel bad about yourself. It is relentless, always telling you that you must try harder to be better because you are never good enough. It is a harsh critic who constantly reprimands you for eating too much or for eating the wrong thing. It criticizes what you say, how you look, and what you do.

The voice in your heart, on the other hand, is the soft, gentle one that begs you to take care of yourself. It is the one that encourages you to stay on track, and reminds you that you are doing your best. It always knows what is best for you. Sometimes this is experienced as a strong pull either to do or not do something. For example, you may suddenly feel an intense need to challenge yourself in some way by expanding your nutritional plan, or by exploring a more difficult topic in therapy. Other times you may feel repelled from things, such as limiting the amount of time you spend with certain people. In either situation, your inner voice will guide you towards health.

You might need help discriminating between the voices of your inner critic and your heart, especially in the early stages of recovery. For example, you may want to exercise more but feel that somehow you shouldn't. One voice tells you that exercise is healthy and good for you, the other suggests that the extra calorie-burning will not help your recovery. In the past, you gave in to the anorexic drive to work out, but now you want to do what is best for you. A trusted friend, family member or therapist may be able to help you figure this out until you can recognize your loving voice on your own.

Sometimes, your heart guides you by sending signals to you through your body. In order to follow its guidance you need to be tuned in to it, and you need to know how to interpret those signals. Begin by paying attention to how you feel when you think about a certain topic. Experiencing stress and tightness in your chest, back, neck, or stomach is a signal from your heart that indicates that that particular thing is not good for you. The tightness is your heart saying, "No." Otherwise, you're probably on the right track. If you are breathing comfortably and your body is more at ease, your inner guidance is saying, "Yes." That is the feeling to follow.

Hearing the voice in your heart is only part of the connection; making the commitment to follow its guidance is also necessary. This is where willingness and courage come in. Many of the thoughts, feelings, and behaviors associated with anorexia are harmful, and your inner voice will urge you to make the proper changes. Trust that what your heart is telling you to do is exactly what you need.

Hearing and honoring the voice in your heart is a skill that needs to be developed. Whenever you find yourself feeling off-center or overly critical, make it a point to stop and find a quiet spot to check in with your heart. Actually stop and sit! This will help bring you back to center so you can refocus your intent. Also, set aside quiet time each day to make this connection through meditation, prayer, inspirational reading, uplifting music, being in nature, or some other activity that quiets your mind and touches your heart. Even at a distant murmur, your inner voice is there. Take the time to listen.

I have spent so much of my life listening to people tell me that I am wrong and that I don't know what I am talking about that it has made it really hard for me to trust myself. When I am able to let myself follow my instincts, I am amazed at how accurate they really are. Right now I am working on trying to follow them as much as possible.

Inner guidance is an amazingly accurate thing when you are connected to it. It's something like having an inner compass. If you are connected to it and following it, you'll always be headed in the right direction. In the beginning, I had to write things down on paper and study them to see if it was anorexia talking or my inner self. It was an intellectual exercise at first. I was so used to hearing anorexia and listening to it, that it was hard to hear another voice. But that other voice was and continues to be there.

People can tell you what to do all through recovery, but I have learned that if it doesn't feel right in my heart, it isn't going to work.

The voice in my heart is driven by love. It has my best interest in mind and it loves me unconditionally. It was hard for me to follow, I think, because I didn't believe I deserved that. The trick was to just follow it anyway.

CHAPTER 4

Get Support

While no one can walk the road to recovery for you, it is good to remember that you do not have to walk it alone. Actually, getting support is an important recovery tool, because anorexia is such an isolating disease. Sufferers compete for the thinnest body and the highest degree of self-sufficiency. Their minds are constantly spinning with thoughts of food, low self-esteem, and the fear of losing control. They are cut off from their own bodies, even as they approach starvation. Their limited world of anorexia pushes them increasingly into isolation, and they withdraw from normal social life.

Entering into safe relationships with family, friends, or professional caregivers is a way to break through this isolation. In a trusting relationship, you are assured attention and respect. You learn to express your thoughts and feelings honestly, without the fear of being judged or rejected. Ultimately, you will discover that the rewards of connecting with people who care about you far outweigh the loneliness of anorexia.

You may be embarrassed to ask for support, or fear that once you open up, people may try to make you do something before you are ready. Perhaps you have been hurt in a past relationship, which makes you distrust others, or you just don't feel good enough

about yourself to share. But these feelings and beliefs are perpetu-
ating your anorexia. Gather your willingness and courage to seek
out support, and you will discover that a healthy relationship is
fulfilling in a way that an obsession with food is not.

Remember that whatever support you choose—family, friends,
professionals, programs or other avenues—you deserve to be respected in all of your relationships. The connections you make
with others should be empowering and helpful, and if they aren't,
assert your needs and change the situation.

Professional Help: The Treatment Team

Due to the complexity and seriousness of anorexia, we strongly
suggest that individuals with anorexia seek help from professionals who have training and experience in the treatment of eating
disorders. Many people opt to work with a "treatment team" which
is a combination of professionals who work together to provide
the most comprehensive support available. A treatment team
commonly consists of any combination of the following: medical doctors, psychiatrists, therapists, nutritionists, dietitians, and
social workers.

The relationship with your doctors and other team members
should be characterized by mutual respect. You should feel comfortable asking questions, and they should answer honestly and
with compassion. When you begin your search for potential therapists and physicians, set up interviews. Come prepared with a list
of questions and concerns, and note how they reply. This is a time
when it is especially valuable to pay attention to your inner voice. If
you feel good around someone, believe that they are knowledgeable
about treating anorexia, find their office inviting, and would like

them to work with you on your recovery, go for it! Otherwise, continue your search until you find someone that you like.

There are numerous ways to find eating disorders professionals. Local help is available in most areas through referrals from a family physician, school counseling center, or local hospital. Check the yellow pages of your telephone book (try "Therapists" or "Psychologists") or search the Internet. Some non-profit eating disorders associations (listed in "Resources") provide referrals. Also, there are several respected inpatient facilities that specialize in eating disorders which accept patients from all over the country. Of course, you will want to contact your health insurance provider to find out what coverage is included with your policy. In some cases, you might expect to have out-of-pocket expenses— but there's no better investment than in your long-term health and happiness.

Here's a breakdown of the components of a treatment team:

Medical Management

We highly recommended that you get a complete physical exam when you begin your recovery process, and retain a medical doctor as part of your treatment team, even as you get better. An M.D. can monitor your overall health and help you to gauge your progress. As we pointed out earlier, there are many potential medical problems associated with anorexia, and with the support of an understanding and knowledgeable doctor, you can address those that apply to you.

Most physicians who work with anorexics are empathic, compassionate people who understand that the issues that brought you to them are complex. Many will generously offer you words of hope and encouragement. Even though you may feel embarrassed talking about your symptoms at first, be as honest as you can so that your doctor can fully utilize his or her abilities. If at any time you do become medically unstable, your doctor should clearly explain the situation to you in understandable terms. For instance, a steadily decreasing potassium level is something about which your doctor will caution you. He or she will let you know what your level is now, how fast it is decreasing, and at what point you may need supplements or even hospitalization. Outlining your current situation and its risks, they will recommend a specific course of action to take in order to safeguard your life.

Psychiatrists are medical doctors who are also therapists. They can prescribe medication, if indicated, as well as provide therapy. Usually a psychiatric assessment is done in the early stages of recovery from any eating disorder, but in many cases psychiatrists will suggest a psychologist or counselor as your ongoing therapist.

In addition to having physical and psychological checkups, you should also be seen by a dentist, particularly if you have been vomiting.

My medical doctor is very supportive, whereas others have made me feel like a hypochondriac. She understands that I have a chemical imbalance and wants to help me find the right medication. She always says that she respects me for how hard I am trying to get better.

I always felt like my doctor cared about me and what happened to me. That made all the difference in the world. I felt like I mattered, and that fueled my desire to recover.

My doctor was compassionate and understanding. He explained the consequences of my anorexia, but he never judged me.

Therapy

Professional therapy is usually the most important component of recovery from an eating disorder. For many anorexics, it is the first and sometimes only place that they can be heard, supported, and validated.

There are many types of therapists and a wide variety of approaches. A therapist can be a psychologist, marriage and family counselor, school counselor, social worker, or other trained professional. Your specific situation and the therapist's training and orientation will dictate the therapeutic approach.

Most eating disorders therapy includes: one-on-one psychotherapy; psychoeducation about sociocultural, historical, feminist, and medical issues; nutritional counseling; drug treatment; group sessions; family or couples therapy; and body-image work. Alternative approaches include experiential therapies such as art or movement therapy and psychodrama; body work, such as therapeutic touch; the use of hypnosis; psychospiritual explorations; and physically-challenging empowering techniques such as wilderness courses.

If all of this seems overwhelming to you, relax. Remember that your recovery and the therapeutic process takes time. You will be exposed to these approaches and new support at a rate that your primary therapist thinks you can handle. Everyone goes through recovery at their own pace, and you will not be pushed beyond your capacity; but, recovery from an eating disorder is hard work. Be willing to extend yourself at times and try new things.

In choosing a therapist, seek out someone who has at least some experience working with eating disorders. Make sure that you find a person with whom you feel comfortable expressing yourself, because during the course of therapy you will need to address your deepest feelings as well as the difficult circumstances that led to and now maintain your anorexia.

Plan on spending the first few sessions getting acquainted with each other. Don't expect to share your deepest secrets right away. Some things may be too painful to admit to yourself, let alone say out loud to someone you have just met. Be patient and gentle with yourself, and give your relationship with your therapist time to develop. Honor your process and your own inner unfolding; it has its own rhythm for a reason. If, after several sessions, you are not yet comfortable with your therapist, or if things feel generally "wrong," listen to that inner voice. You may not be a good match, and you should consider finding someone else.

Remember that no treatment professional has all the answers or is right all the time. They may occasionally misinterpret something that you say or give you feedback that is off the mark. Good clinicians will rely on you to provide them with feedback and suggestions about what helps and what doesn't.

Therapy has been an integral part of my healing. It has helped me explore my life, myself, and my perceptions of both. In fact, it has been a crucial part of discovering who I am. It isn't always easy, but I believe my recovery and my health depends on my persevering in my therapy.

The relationship I have with my therapist took time and effort to develop. It still takes time and nurturing to maintain. It isn't a relationship that comes with ease, at least it didn't for me. But it's worth all the effort!

I have had several therapists, each of which has helped me in a different way. Leaving them to go on to the next was always hard because we had shared so much. A good therapist will even help you leave them!

Nutritional Counseling

A nutritionist or registered dietitian offers very specific support—helping you normalize your eating, while educating you about food and your body's nutritional needs. Taking into consideration your food preferences and weight restoration needs, they will develop a customized food plan that is both acceptable and tolerable to you. Meeting at regular intervals, you can discuss your progress, talk about specific concerns, and create strategies to conquer the problems you may be having with particular meals or foods. For most anorexics, normalizing their eating is an uncomfortable process, and nutritional counseling often makes it more manageable.

As with the other members of your treatment team, you should feel comfortable asking questions about specific food fears, weight gain, and healthy eating. Keep in mind that most nutritionists are not trained to discuss the personal, underlying issues of an eating disorder; these are normally reserved for sessions with your therapist.

My nutritionist guaranteed that I wouldn't get fat, so I wasn't too afraid to gain the weight. She gave me a feeling of control, even though she was the one in charge! She worked around my food idiosyncrasies so that I would succeed.

My nutritionist was one of my greatest allies. He worked closely with me to develop a plan that I could follow. I was never someone who could eat "three square meals" but he explained that was okay. We made up a plan for me to eat little meals throughout the day, which worked well.

My dietician taught me about my body's needs and how to eat for optimal health and well-being. Now, I am aware of how good I feel and how much energy I have.

Treatment Programs

Specialized eating disorders treatment programs are available at some hospitals. There are also facilities specifically dedicated to eating disorders that accept patients from all over the world (see "Resources"). These facilities have a variety of care levels, including:

• Inpatient—Patients live at the facility around-the-clock for an extended period, ranging from a couple of weeks to several months. Settings vary from hospital wards to dormitories to group houses. Inpatient is the preferred treatment for those with medical complications, or for those needing constant supervision.

• Residential—Patients stay in a dorm-like setting with somewhat less supervision than an inpatient unit. The participation level is about the same. Inpatients commonly graduate to a residential program, or in some situations when space is not available for inpatient services, residential treatment is chosen.

- Day-hospital—Participants report to the facility each morning, stay all day, and return home in the evening. They take full advantage of treatment without the costs of housing.

- Outpatient—Individuals meet with treatment team members and groups on a scheduled basis while continuing with their normal living routine.

Most treatment programs use a multidimensional approach with staffs generally consisting of psychologists, psychiatrists, internists, social workers, nutritionists, and sometimes recreational, physical and occupational therapists, as well. Most programs assign a case manager or treatment coordinator to keep track of scheduling and communication needs.

A typical day at a treatment facility will include individual therapy sessions, meetings with nutritionists, appointments with physicians, support groups and educational classes, and structured meals. Groups and classes might cover such areas as: body image, stress management, food and relationships, eating disorders coping skills, nutrition education, relapse prevention, anger management, women's issues, assertiveness training, art or music therapy, and expressive writing therapy.

Being surrounded by others who share your experience is an important aspect of being in a treatment program. Your peers will understand you in ways that friends and family members may not. They can help you realize that you are not alone. Hearing others openly discuss their behaviors and thinking patterns may help alleviate your fears and embarrassment, which will allow you to talk more openly. Supporting others in their recoveries can also be a way for you to feel good about yourself.

Most programs require that patients eat together in a supportive environment, commonly called "supervised meals." Because mealtimes tend to be highly emotional events, staff members are present to maintain a safe, low-stress environment. Certain topics are restricted from discussion, such as calories, exercise, weight, and diets. Staff members are available to offer immediate assistance to anyone struggling with high anxiety. Often, group members discover feelings of camaraderie at mealtime, and a palpable feeling of "You can do it" support is sometimes present at the table. Meals are followed by activities planned to prevent purging and to distract or address discomfort.

The intense support offered by dedicated treatment programs is valuable for numerous reasons. Although medical stabilization may be the most obvious, people also enter programs to get extra support during a crisis period, to renew motivation that has waned, to learn new skills, and to identify issues which need to be addressed. They act as springboards to hurdle the obstacles on the road to recovery by providing knowledgeable support and encouragement, thereby increasing the chances of a full recovery.

Entering a treatment facility was one of the most important things I did for my recovery. It taught me how to focus, identify the areas I needed to work on, and set reasonable, realistic goals for myself.

My treatment program helped me with all aspects of my recovery. It helped me pace my work so that I didn't get too overwhelmed. I wouldn't say that the program cured me, but it certainly got me on the right track.

The best thing was having a lot of support right there whenever I needed it. It also made me feel good to lend support to other people.

Family and Loved Ones

If you live with your parents and siblings or have a spouse or significant other, and if they are open to supporting you, recovery can be a shared experience at home and in family therapy. Your family and loved ones care about your health and happiness; at times, they may even be more committed to your recovery than you are! Talk to them about your concerns, and honor theirs, as well. Be open to a change in your relationship as you commit to this difficult journey together. There are tremendous growth opportunities here for everyone involved.

Also, educating all members of your household about eating disorders is important. Using resources such as books, information from national eating disorder organizations, and professional guidance, you can explore how you are going to work together towards your recovery goals. You will need to address both everyday concerns as well as more general issues, from discovering new ways of dealing with food choices to healthier ways of communicating. This is the time for everyone to look at their own personal strengths and weaknesses; to confront their prejudices on topics such as cultural pressures to be thin, emerging sexuality, and intimacy; and to re-examine family rules and values.

Family support can take different forms—a brainstorming session of recovery ideas, a loved one listening to your deepest thoughts and feelings, or cooperation in meal planning and food preparation. Support can be financial, providing for professional treatment. A supportive sibling might take a quiet walk with you, helping you to keep from breaking into an obsessive exercise binge. Or an anorexic's father might help by telling his daughter that he loves her regardless of her size and weight. Find out what works together, and remember that the more support you are willing to accept, the more help you will receive.

Keep in mind that not all families are able to be supportive. There may be obvious limits due to distance or death, and sometimes family members—even with good intentions—are emotionally incapable. They may be overly controlling or judgmental, and cannot grasp or hear your concerns. If your family is more of the problem than the solution, you might need to distance yourself and look for support elsewhere. Explain why you are excluding them, if that's possible, because sometimes the truth can bring you closer, even if it hurts. Whether they are going to support you or not, it is valuable to recognize their influence.

It has been both good and bad for me to include my family—a double-edged sword. On the one hand, I felt a lot closer to my husband when he was going to family therapy with me, but on the other, he wanted more results. I felt a lot of pressure to hurry up and get well.

My sisters and brother went to therapy with me, but it didn't feel right to have them in the therapeutic role. Now they are acting like they used to, but they want me to take more responsibility for what I need. If something they say or do bothers me, I am supposed to speak up. This means that I have to be more assertive, which is hard, but good for me.

My boyfriend, who encouraged me and stood by me, is now my husband. He knows all my deep, dark secrets. He even went to therapy with me to try and understand what I was going through.

Other Support

There are many other obvious, and perhaps not so obvious, places to find support. Certainly, good friends will be there for you, as might others like a special teacher, a spiritual advisor, or someone else who has recovered. You can even get encouragement from taking your dog for a walk or talking to your cat. They won't have anything to say in response, but sometimes a good listener is better than a talker anyway! Besides, they love you unconditionally.

The point here is not *who* you find to help you, but rather that you realize that you do not need to face recovery alone. In fact, you *cannot* do it alone; thinking that you can is part of your anorexia. Breaking through your isolation and entering authentic, supportive relationships is one of the most important healing steps you can take.

Individuals who have recovered from anorexia make particularly good support choices. Being in the presence of someone who is no longer tortured by obsessive thoughts of food and weight, *but who knows exactly what that feels like*, is a tremendously powerful and reassuring experience. Spending time with someone who has recovered is like looking hope directly in the eye. You can sit with them and say to yourself, "This person was once just like I am, and now she is really okay!" This relationship can makes recovery feel much more tangible, much more possible.

A recovered mentor will try to answer all your questions about recovery. He or she hurdled the same kinds of obstacles you are facing now, and will be able provide you with unique and invaluable insights. In addition to offering wisdom and understanding, a recovered person can model the healthy behaviors and new ways of thinking that you are trying so hard to acquire. Spending time with people who are taking care of themselves will reinforce your new behaviors, making it easier for you to stick with them. Many eating disorder organizations, hospitals, colleges, high schools, and women's organizations sponsor panels of recovered women who will speak to various audiences. These groups can refer you to someone, as can your therapist.

Recovered people lend a unique kind of hope. They can remove doubts like no one else can. They can say, "Oh yeah, I've been there. Look at where you can go!" And suddenly it seems possible.

After I hear someone speak about their recovery from anorexia, I feel really motivated. I work harder and feel more hopeful. I wish there was a recovered person I could just hang out with all day, everyday, until I'm fully there.

Talking on a regular basis to a friend who had recovered was a key factor in my ability to conquer my food and weight-related fears. It helped me take risks and finally start to trust my body.

When I was in the hospital, my biggest fear was that my night-mares and flashbacks of abuse were going to get worse. I missed my cat and how she made me feel so safe and loved.

Currently I am seeing a counselor at school, and am devoted to getting well. She gave me a book on eating disorders that seemed to describe me perfectly. It gave me hope.

CHAPTER 5

What Has Worked for Many

While we highly recommend getting professional help for anorexia, we also feel that there is a lot of work that can be done on one's own, outside of the treatment setting. For this reason, we offer this "hands-on" chapter, with discussions, exercises, and suggestions for activities that you can use to foster your own recovery. Each section explores one topic and ends with quotes from other recovering and recovered anorexics. Not all topics will relate directly to you, but many will. Be creative with your recovery process. The suggestions are just that—suggestions. Use them in a way that feels best to *you*, because, in the end, *you* are your own best teacher.

This chapter will provide you with an opportunity to examine your disorder—to investigate why you have it, to understand what currently supports it, and also to learn how to be happy and fulfilled without it. We know that this process can be frightening and overwhelming; we know because we have been through it. Commend yourself for doing this work. You are a warrior, and these are the ways of a warrior.

The following sections in this chapter are filled with ideas, exercises, and insights from people who have recovered from anorexia nervosa:

SECTIONS IN CHAPTER 5

- Get to Know Yourself
- Journal Writing
- Identify Goals
- Challenge Cultural Influences
- Have Compassion
- Change Your Mind
- Feel Your Feelings
- Be Gentle with Your Pain
- Body Image Work
- Relaxation
- Strengthen Your Boundaries
- Cultivate Relationships
- Spiritual Pursuits
- Let Go
- Express Yourself
- Focus on Recovery

Get to Know Yourself

As you begin to let go of the behaviors that anorexia so rigidly dictates, you may suddenly realize that you do not know who you are. Many people say that because they have identified with anorexia for so long, they feel as though they are losing their own selves. This can be a lonely experience. But once you begin your recovery, you will realize that *it's you that you are lonely for.*

By practicing the rigid behaviors that dominate your days and occupy your thoughts, anorexia separates you from your inner self. You no longer have the ability to dream because your only dream is to be thinner. You no longer know how to play and laugh, because losing weight is serious business. You no longer know who you are on the inside, because all your attention is focused on external standards of beauty and success.

Essential to recovery from an eating disorder is getting to know who you are *on the inside*. This means spending time investigating your thoughts, feelings, beliefs, joys, pains, and all else that makes up your inner life. You can do this in many ways, some of which are suggested in this chapter, and others which you can create on your own.

Little by little, as you get to know yourself, you will come to know that there is so much more to you than the size of your body. You will discover that within your heart is a loving, creative, wise, strong, and beautiful person waiting to be found. There is also more behind your disorder than your fear of fat, such as your family history, your social and cultural environment, and the range of your personal experiences. But anorexia prevents you from knowing this by preoccupying you with rules, rituals, and external standards. True validation, you will discover, can only be found by looking inward. The strength to overcome this illness is within you. Take the time to discover who you *really* are. Remember that all relationships require time and nurturing in order to develop, and the relationship you have with yourself is no different.

Write Your Story

Write the story of your life, with particular emphasis on the events that were happening when you first became self-conscious of your body. Then explore in detail what those events meant to you and how they made you feel. This exercise can take days or even months, as you get to know yourself better in the course of your recovery. Perhaps draw a time line marking important events. Also, plot a family tree. Note individual problems and look for patterns. Can you find your body type? Are there others in your family who have problems with food and weight, or related problems like depression, alcoholism, or social avoidance? Explore in detail whatever comes to mind in order to get to know yourself and understand how anorexia has helped you cope.

I know myself a lot better than I used to. Now I know that the past had nothing to do with me, it had to do with the fact that my parents didn't know how to bring up someone from a different culture. I'm an adopted Native American.

I now know that I am not a bad person. I am actually kind, compassionate, smart, funny, and extremely giving. Sometimes I'm mouthy, too, and that's a good thing!

I realized that my food issue was the big "fogger" for what was really going on in my life, I didn't know if I'd make it through . . . I mean, who was I going to be . . . who was I?

Journal Writing

Writing in a journal is possibly the most widely-used recovery tool. Because it is for your eyes only, your journal is a sacred, safe place to express all your thoughts and feelings without the fear of being exposed. Consistently writing your truth in a journal is potentially the most powerful process of your entire recovery. For this reason, we recommend that you write at least once every day.

Once you begin "talking" openly and honestly with yourself, you'll want to check in regularly. When you feel anxious, lonely, frightened or overwhelmed, remember that your journal is a trusted friend to whom you can turn. It is also a perfect place to savor joyful moments and triumphs, and to examine past events that have influenced the way you now treat yourself. Keep your journal with you so you will always have a "friend" within reach.

Use your journal for exploring issues. One good question is, *What are you recovering to?* Something will have to take the place of the anorexia when it is gone. What will that be? It is a lot easier to know what you *don't* want in your life, but you must give some consideration to what you *do* want, for instance: healthy coping skills, nurturing relationships, gentle self-respect, etc. Make a list, knowing that it will be unique to you. Then, with your list in front of you, ask that this list come true. Repeat this process throughout your recovery, as your goals will change as you grow. Asking for what you want will not only point you towards your future, but it will also help you let go of the past.

Here are more suggested writing assignments:

TOPICS FOR WRITTEN EXPLORATION

• Write one sentence each about five or ten good things in your life.

• Describe one of the happiest moments of your life. Try to remember why you felt so good about yourself at that time. Hold on to those good feelings for the rest of the day.

• List ten people you admire (five you personally know and five you know from society or history). What attributes do they have that you admire? List your attributes. Which ones do you admire in yourself?

• Pick one family member, and write in-depth about your impressions of them as well as your relationship with them. Describe some dramatic experiences you had together. Why were those events so relevant, and how did they make you feel? Choose another family member on another writing occasion.

• Make a list of 5-10 myths and 5-10 rules thaty you want to change. A myth may be something like, "Skinny people are happier," and a rule might be, "If I eat dessert, I have to do 100 situps."

• Make lists of short-term and long-term goals. Cross out any entries that have to do with losing weight, burning calories, etc.

• What can you do to become more self loving?

The following are suggested topics to explore from the book *Anorexia Nervosa: The Wish to Change* (Crisp 1996):

MORE TOPICS . . .

- The meaning of my shape to me
- My family's use of avoidance to deal with conflict
- My use of avoidance to deal with conflict
- My relationship with authority
- My sense of self; social and sexual
- My impulses and the way I manage them
- My present or future career; why I have chosen it

Use your journal to practice new ways of thinking. When you write, you will discover new ways of coping. Affirm healthy thoughts, and write even things that you do not yet know to be true. Regularly affirming these things will help you to know their truth. Here are some good affirmations; come up with more of your own:

AFFIRMATIONS

- I can eat without fear!
- Every day, in every way, I'm getting better and better.
- My weight has nothing to do with my worth.
- I deserve good things.
- I trust the Universe.
- I am grateful for my life.
- People care about me.
- I have a good heart.
- My body takes good care of me.

- I allow myself to feel.
- I need to listen to my heart and honor my process.
- I am love.

I write in my journal every day without fail. It helps me stay connected to myself and my feelings. I know from experience that when I feel disconnected from myself, I am likely to get into trouble.

I love my journal. I can write what I can't say. Sometimes I share my writing with my therapist and we use it as a starting point for sessions.

My journal is a tremendous outlet to write about my feelings, memories, and experiences, both good and bad. If there is a particular memory that really bothers me, sometimes writing it in my journal makes it possible to move on for awhile until I can talk about it in therapy. It's like "putting" the thought someplace, which really helps.

Identify Goals

Life doesn't get put on hold once you make the decision to recover; there will always be issues that demand your time and attention. Scheduling time each day to identify goals and plan strategies to reach them is an effective way to ensure that your recovery does not get lost or put on hold amidst the hustle and bustle of everyday life.

In your journal or in a separate goals notebook, identify at least one goal for each day, either short-term or long-term. Underneath your goal or goals, write down strategies which will help you handle any problems or difficult feelings that might arise as you strive to reach them. Also identify resources that you might be able to use for support. For example, if your goal is to complete all meals, some strategies might be affirmations or breathing exercises to help with the anxiety, setting the table nicely, or saying a prayer before the meal. You could call a friend before you begin, or have someone sit with you. The more strategies you have, the better—they will help you stay focused and motivated. Finally, at the end of the day, set aside time to review the results. Were you able to achieve your goal? Did your strategies help? How do you feel about your goal? What else might you try?

Keeping track of your goals and strategies takes conscious thought and work. Sometimes you may really have to push yourself. Give yourself rewards for every success. Go over your goal experiences with your therapist or support person to help you stay committed to this learning process. You will find that recording and working on concrete goals is a valuable tool that is well worth the effort. Here are some areas for improvement (Crisp p.54):

AREAS FOR IMPROVEMENT

- Asserting myself
- Being spontaneous
- Communicating
- Decision making
- Eating with others
- Expression of feelings
- Feeling in charge of myself
- Having fun
- Indulging myself

- Loving others
- My self-esteem
- Owning my sexuality
- Socializing
- Thinking of others
- Trusting others

Having a distinct goal each day reminded me that I was working on my recovery one piece at a time. I knew I didn't have to do everything all at once.

I think it is important not to label your goals as successes or failures. If you meet a goal one day, congratulate yourself; otherwise, just keep working on it. The object isn't to beat yourself up, it is to move forward.

One of my goals was to eat one "forbidden" food every day without guilt. This was one of the hardest things I had to do.

Challenge Cultural Influences

While there are many personal issues to explore in recovery, there are also cultural factors which contribute to your eating disorder.

First, and perhaps most obvious, is the fact that we live in a culture that worships thinness. This is not news for anyone, least of all people who suffer from anorexia. A thin body is equated with health, happiness, success, intelligence, sexuality and a host of other positives. The media is saturated by images of thin models conveying this message. Billions of dollars every year are spent by the diet, fashion, and beauty industries to convince women, and increasing numbers of men, to be different from the way they naturally are—and especially to be thin. This obsession has made us think that our appearance is more important than what we think, do, or feel, and that thinness is a means to success and power. This has created fertile ground for eating disorders.

The flip side to this obsession with thinness is our hatred of fat, which is falsely equated with disease, stupidity, lack of will-power, failure, and other negatives. Again, the media stereotypes fat people in these ways. While we have become more accepting of others regardless of their race, religion, or gender, weight prejudice is widespread and generally accepted. In the face of horrible discrimination, it is not surprising that 90% of women have dieted, or that the most radical of those dieters— anorex-ics—fear weight gain more than anything. But who wants to live their lives filled with hatred and fear? The restrictions of forced thinness are simply not worth the effort, which W. Charisse Goodman points out in *The Invisible Woman: Confronting Weight Prejudice in America,*

> Imagine intentionally detaching all moral content from the acts of eating and exercising. Eventually the automatic anxiety and self-reproach fade away, and your relationship with food be-comes more relaxed. You and you alone are in complete con-trol of your body. You find better things to do besides worrying about food and avoiding (or being preoccupied with) mirror images. You begin to regain the energy that has been drained by self-hatred and unrealistic expectations. (p. 181)

Also, while strides have been made in the area of women's rights, ours is a still a predominately male-dominated culture.

Women are generally paid less than men, rarely attain the highest political or corporate positions, are subjected to harassment and violence, and are inescapably viewed as sexual objects. Even as they break equality barriers, they continue to feel the pressure to put others first, not be too needy, and make themselves agreeable to men. An eating disorder can be a way to cope with the fear and lack of fulfillment that comes from being devalued and treated as a sexual object or second-class citizen.

What's more, our culture as a whole embodies masculine traits like competitiveness, independence, and aggression. This leaves many women, who are naturally more nurturing, interdependent, and cooperative, feeling invalidated and out-of-place. An eating disorder can be a way to avoid the confusion of what it means to be a woman in a such a male-oriented environment. Men who develop anorexia—whether heterosexual or homosexual—are typically more sensitive than the "average" male, and they, too, use their eating disorder to retreat from such a hostile society.

As Kim Chernin wrote in her classic book, *The Obsession: Reflections on the Tyranny of Slenderness*,

> A woman obsessed with the size of her body, wishing to make her breasts and thighs and hips and belly smaller and less apparent, may be expressing the fact that she feels uncomfortable being female in this culture. (p. 2)

Unfortunately, even though society is slowly evolving, we cannot force social change. Despite decades of advocacy, activists in the women's movement and size-acceptance field and eating disorders educators have made minimal progress towards ending our unreasonable standards of beauty and limited gender roles.

However, we can individually choose to rise above cultural oppression. In fact, your recovery mandates that you do so.

NINE WAYS TO CHALLENGE CULTURAL INFLUENCES

- Dieting is a form of oppression; do not diet!

- Notice how television stereotypes people according to weight, and turn off those kinds of shows.

- Tear out and discard magazine photos of skinny women. How many pictures of women are left?

- Write letters to advertisers and manufacturers that promote values of thinness. Tell them how they've contributed to your anorexia.

- Respect people without regard to their size.

- Take the energy that you spend on your obsession with food and weight, and funnel it in a more productive direction.

- Don't tolerate negative comments that others make about weight.

- Get involved with, or financially support, organizations that promote size acceptance or eating disorders prevention.

- Reject your fear of fat.

Magazines and TV shows make you think that you have to be thin. If you are anything larger, you are unacceptable. I don't buy magazines any more.

There's so much pressure to perform, to compete with other people—physically, mentally, and emotionally. It's crazy. Now, I don't worry about being thinner or more perfect. I'm just me.

Women (and men!) need to challenge the institutions that keep them from knowing their true worth. We shouldn't be competing, we should be turning to each other!

Have Compassion

Most recovered anorexics agree that finding compassion for themselves was what allowed recovery to begin, progress, and finally stick for good. Learning to love and care for yourself is a deliberate process that requires you to ask and answer many painful questions, while challenging your perceptions about yourself and the world around you. Steadfastly walking this rewarding path of introspection, however, will lead you from self-hate to self-acceptance and eventually to self-love.

Learning to treat yourself with compassion is no simple task. It is particularly difficult if you have been treated harshly or thought poorly of yourself for most of your life. You may not believe that you deserve to be treated well by anyone—especially yourself. You may not even feel that you deserve to be happy! These are not easy beliefs to overcome, but you *must* in order to heal.

Being compassionate with yourself may mean different things at different times. It might mean letting yourself cry, or forcing yourself to get up and move despite the pain. It might mean setting gentle but firm boundaries or allowing yourself more freedom. It might mean taking risks. Always, though, being compassionate means accepting yourself unconditionally. Anorexia was the best that you could do in order to survive; but now, with new understanding and determination, you can do better. You can treat yourself with love and respect, affirming that you are worth every positive step you take.

At times you may think that you are not making as much progress as you would like, but learning to care about yourself is a process with its own ebb and flow. Do not let yourself become discouraged. Once you have experienced compassion for yourself, you can never permanently lose it. Throughout your recovery, remind yourself to accept where you are. Trust that in allowing your recovery to take its own unique shape, you are caring about yourself in a new way.

One exercise for practicing compassion is to close your eyes and imagine what caring about yourself "looks like." How do you start and end your day? Be descriptive, use details. Feel yourself experiencing a full day of compassionate thoughts, words and actions. Really enjoy this experience. When you can truly see the love as it plays out in everyday experiences, you will manifest the ensuing results of peace and joy.

Now, try something a bit more active. Collect pictures of yourself as a child. As vividly as you can, imagine spending a day with this child. Where do you take her? To the park for a swing fest? On a hike with a picnic lunch? To the ice-cream shop for a scoop of peppermint stick? Spend some time, maybe every day for one week, with a different photo. Eventually you will come to recognize that the child in those pictures is really yourself—worthy of all good things.

When I first started to really experience love for myself, I found it to be bittersweet. There was joy as I began to appreciate myself as a valuable, lovable being. But there was also grief. It's amazing how

*much old injustices and injuries hurt when you finally love your-
self. My compassion for myself is what assures me that I will get
through it.*

*Loving myself was definitely the key to my recovery. It's true, you
can't hurt something or someone you love.*

Change Your Mind

People with eating disorders are locked into negative thinking
patterns and beliefs. Like water flowing down a hillside, their
thoughts follow the same lines day after day, becoming deeply
ingrained. In your recovery from anorexia, you must become aware
of, and fight to change, these patterns, because they are perpetu-
ating your illness.

First, however, you must begin to eat healthfully, because your
brain does not function properly when you are malnourished. Im-
paired serotonin levels due to anorexia can cause obsessional symptoms, anxiety, low moods, inhibition, and drowsiness. (Zerbe p.
275) These problems can seriously affect all of your thinking. But as
you begin to allow your body to heal, you will have a clearer mind
and be better able to make changes in how you think.

The next step is to become aware of your thoughts. This may
seem like a silly idea, but have you ever *thought* about what you
think? If you were able to step back and *look* at your thoughts, as
an objective observer, you might discover that you are playing
destructive "tapes" over and over. This inner chatter goes on constantly, spinning from one topic to another, affecting everything
you feel and do. For this reason, an important job in recovery is to
clearly decipher those internal "tapes" so you can transform them—

from a negative into a positive force for change. Simply put, to get to self-love, you must first recognize self-hate.

A few examples of negative thinking patterns are:

- **Seeing everything as black or white.**

Food becomes good or bad; weight gain equals obesity. You *always* look in the full-length mirror, but *never* walk when you can run, etc.

- **Magnifying the negatives.**

Filtering out the positives, and letting only the negatives through. Minor problems are seen as catastrophes, and comments get blown out of proportion. If you see an increase on the scale, the day is ruined. If someone disagrees with an opinion, you think they hate you.

- **Taking everything personally.**

Thinking that the world revolves around you. If you see a picture in a magazine, you compare whether or not you are thinner. You feel guilty over matters that often have nothing to do with you. You may feel that people are judging you or that the world is against you. Relationships are sometimes one-sided, because people tiptoe around you, afraid of how you might react.

- **The "shoulds."**

Having rigid rules about how you and others should act. This can lead you to place unreasonable demands on yourself like, "I should not express anger," or "I should only eat carrot sticks for lunch." The "shoulds" make you think that you control things that might very well be out of your control.

These tapes, in a way, define your existence. What you *think* becomes your reality. What you think also manifests in your life; it is the bridge between you and the outside world. So, if you think that you are a bad person, you might think that you don't deserve to eat, and won't. Or, if you think that getting angry will get you in trouble, you might starve your anger. On the other hand, if you think that you can recover from your anorexia, and firmly plant that idea in your every waking and sleeping minute, you will begin to get better. *What you think has the power to change your life.*

Changing your mind is not as simple as it sounds, however. Saying something new and really believing it to be true are two different matters. But the simple act of substituting positive thoughts for negative ones can affect you on a much deeper level, and so you must force yourself. First, learn to be aware of the "tapes" you play inside your head. What does your self-talk sound like? Do you really mean to tell yourself that you are lazy, ugly, worthless? Wouldn't it feel better to affirm that you are valuable, worthy, beautiful, and one of God's perfect creations?

CHANGING YOUR MIND

- Instead of leaving your thoughts on automatic, recognize and stop the negatives.

- Practice different, more positive self-talk through speaking and writing.

- Question your beliefs. When you discover that old ones do not apply to your present life, create new ones.

- Have discussions with other people about what they believe.

- Be open to constructive criticism.

- Redirect or reframe negative statements. Say out

loud, "I am a great person," even if you don't believe it 100%.

• Above all, take quiet time to give your mind a rest and get "beyond" the chatter. When you quiet your mind, you can more easily hear the voice in your heart.

Self-acceptance exercise:

Take an entire day to accept everything about yourself. You may feel that this is ridiculous, but do it anyway. It is just one day. After your morning shower, for example, as you towel off and are getting dressed, take a moment to look in the mirror. If a voice wants to point out flaws, tell it to go away. You are having a *self-acceptance day*. If, later on, you find yourself using words like, "stupid, bad, ugly," stop the thought. Replace it with, "I am bright, good, and beautiful." Repeat affirmative statements, both written and verbal—this act rewrites your internal script. Feel the energy of the words as they sink into your cellular biology—you are changing your thoughts that deeply.

I pretend I have a trap door in my brain and I put all the negative thoughts behind it.

My mind was always on "automatic pilot." My beliefs were all so rigid. One of the hardest things I had to do in my recovery was to slow down, step back, and be aware of my thoughts so I could change them.

Feel Your Feelings

Everyone has feelings and needs ways to cope when those feelings become overwhelming or painful. Anorexia provides this by shifting the focus from feelings to an obsession with food, weight and the body.

Managing feelings is not a skill you are born with, however; it needs to be learned. Perhaps you come from a family that is not comfortable with feelings or that has given you the message that feelings are bad. You may think that feelings are unimportant or that they have the potential for spinning you out of control. If this is the case for you, you may not even be able to identify what the different feelings *are*, much less be able to express them in a healthy way.

This confusion over feelings applies to your relationship with food, as well. Just as you are able to deny your feelings, you are also able to deny your physical hunger. For this reason, identifying and feeling your emotions will help with your food issues. Your inner experiences, your hungers, are all important. They are real. They deserve to be expressed and taken care of. By accepting that feelings and needs are part of our human experience, and by learning how to express them in a safe, trusted environment, you can slowly let them out of hiding. You will no longer need the anorexia to keep them at a safe distance.

One powerful exercise to practice is to go back and remember the difficult emotional times prior to the onset of your anorexia. Using your journal, give yourself blocks of no more than 15 minutes for each memory. Describe in detail the event, and when you are finished, underline with a different color pen the feelings that you wrote down.

For example: "When I was fourteen and playing tennis, I had a coach who told me I was too slow and should lose weight. I was only 120 pounds at the time, so this *confused* me; nobody had ever suggested this before. I also was very *embarrassed*, and grew determined. I did not ever want to be *humiliated* like that again. Now this makes me *mad!* Who was he to say that a healthy, growing teenager needed to lose weight! It also makes me *sad* to realize all the fun I missed out on—the pizza and burger outings, all the carefree times when kids are supposed to be kids."

Work hard to extract the feelings from this event. Perhaps draw pictures to illustrate them or talk to other people who were there to get their impressions. Give your feelings the validation and attention they never got from you or anyone else. Then look at how the eating disorder helped you cope with these feelings. Give yourself the compassion and understanding that you did not have at the time, when you were younger and less equipped to handle such hurtful situations. Now, think about how you want to express your feelings in the present—by avoiding them through anorexia? Or by facing them directly and processing them in a healthy way?

Bring your memory and your new insights to your next therapy session. If you are not working with a therapist, risk sharing with a close friend or trusted relative. If you were fortunate enough to grow up with supportive parents and/or siblings, you will find that sharing these recollections can be quite transformative. Aside from the crucial physical aspects of recovery, learning to acknowledge and deal appropriately with your feelings is probably the most important recovery lesson you will learn.

I am really glad that I recovered. I love being able to feel a whole range of emotions. It makes me feel whole, really human.

Once I identified exactly what my feelings really were, I had to learn to sit with them. I do think that a big part of that is being willing to do it. I had to constantly tell myself to be patient, and remind myself that riding out my rocky feelings was the only way to get better.

I never felt that I had the right to my feelings. I grew up in a family that rejected any kind of human emotion and I learned to internalize everything at a really young age. I'm just now learning to identify and accept my feelings and talk about them. I use affirmations a lot and that helps.

Be Gentle with Your Pain

At some point in your recovery, as you acknowledge the deepest feelings behind your anorexia, you may find yourself in soul-wrenching pain. It is not always possible, at times like this, to laugh or play at the beach in order to cope. This is okay. Be gentle with yourself. Embrace your pain, for it has meaning and can hold the key to your recovery.

In the past, you may have coped with pain by hurting yourself, which gave you some relief from your agony. But we are asking you to try something new. Instead of starving, bingeing, purging or enlisting other self-injurious behavior, promise yourself that you will treat yourself with tenderness. Promise yourself that you will unconditionally accept exactly where you are in your process. Most important of all, do not numb yourself when you are hurting so badly inside. Let your feelings flow, and be there for *you.*

Being gentle is probably something that you instinctually do for others when they are in pain or need comfort. When it comes to yourself, however, you may be at a complete loss as to where or how to begin. Below are some suggestions. Remember that pain is an inevitable part of living and loving in this world. It requires time in order to heal. Pain is also legitimate and has a purpose. You are entitled to your feelings. Embrace them all, even the difficult ones. They are what make you whole.

SOME IDEAS FOR BEING GENTLE WITH PAIN

- Cry, cry and cry some more. Now that your tears are no longer blocked by the dam of anorexia, you are free to let them flow.
- Cuddle with a teddy bear or pet.
- Call someone who will be gentle with you.
- Take a walk. Be present to the beauty of nature.
- Buy or make an encouragement card. Frame it, hang it.
- Listen to music.
- Buy yourself fresh flowers.
- Make art—whatever that means to you.
- Write a poem that describes your feelings.

I take care of myself by holding my big, soft doll, listening to my music, going for a walk, or talking on the phone. These activities make me feel connected and cared for.

When I'm really hurting, I go out into the garden and take care of my plants. That makes me feel connected to nature, and always helps.

Ever since I started volunteering at the nursing home, I became less focused on my own problems. That has helped me to actually feel glad to be alive.

I needed to know that there were legitimate reasons why I felt so bad, and that there were other ways to feel better besides starving myself. Now, I write letters, do needlepoint, and take my dog for long walks.

Body Image Work

Our culture's obsession with appearance has caused a majority of people to distrust and dislike their bodies. Women are supposed to be slim and youthful, men trim and muscular. Even athletes are unhappy with their bodies. Although recent years have seen the introduction of plus-size models, the message that thinner is better is communicated loud and clear through the diet and fashion industries, exercise and fitness products, media images, and advertising. We wrongly equate working on our bodies with good character. Striving for a "perfect body" is the cultural norm.

Unfortunately, there is no such thing as a "perfect body." Standards change, fashions change, even theories on the health risks of large bodies is changing. What's more, trying to have a different body than the one we inherited is an expensive and sometimes risky undertaking. Our bodies want to maintain the weight that nature gave us. The truth is that bodies come in all shapes and sizes, unique to our genes, set point, environment, and age.

Dieting does not work. The vast majority of people who dislike their bodies go on diets, fail, and feel bad about themselves. Others slip into an eating disorder thinking that they have found the solution to the dieting problem. The lucky few realize that their bodies are just fine as they are, and laugh off pressures to be thinner.

Anorexics "succeed" at losing weight when almost everyone else fails. Their bodies become a symbol of their strength, discipline, and ability to acomplish something few can. But, they never attain a "perfect" body either, because thin is never thin enough. And as they lose more and more weight, they lose the cognitive ability to judge themselves accurately. What might have started as a simple diet turned into an addiction, where being thinner is the fix. Furthermore, thinness does not bring all the rewards advertised. Ask yourself: Has being thin brought you the loving relationships, satisfying jobs, and meaningful successes that you expected?

One of the most difficult challenges of recovery is to love your body at any weight. Watching the pounds return and wondering if it will ever stop is terrifying. But remind yourself that your body has a weight range that it *wants* to maintain—your set point. This is the healthiest weight for you, and it is determined by your genes. Trust that your body will take care of this very natural process, and that there is a healthy weight range for you.

Hand-in-hand with reaching your set point is your commitment to defying the cultural influences that led to your problems in the first place. You have to be a revolutionary! The pressure to be thin hurts everyone. Large people are discriminated against, medium-sized people think they need to be smaller, and thin people are afraid of gaining. Everyone is controlling their bodies, when they should be trusting them. Affirm your right to love your body no matter what its size and shape. Communicate that message to others! No one is a better ambassador for size acceptance than someone who has recovered from an eating disorder.

SUGGESTIONS FOR IMPROVING BODY IMAGE

• Talk back to your body critic. Repeat affirmations of your own making like, "My beauty is unique, my body is a gift."

• Notice that everyone's body is different and stop comparing yourself. Neither ultrathin models nor the super heavy should be judged by their bodies, and neither should you.

• Walk and speak with dignity, letting your body language reflect this emerging pride. Be a bigger presence in the world; you deserve to take up space!

• Thank your body for all the good things that it does for you. Pamper it with massages, hot baths, scents, healthy exercise, etc.

• Get to know your body better—wear clothes that fit; appreciate your sexuality.

• Accept compliments graciously, knowing that beauty on the outside reflects beauty on the inside.

• Stop looking in the mirror so often and judging specific parts of your body. See the whole.

• Throw out your scale.

• Read self-help books on improving body image.

• Try guided imagery and visualization techniques.

• Dance, do yoga, experiment with different forms of movement (as opposed to vigorous exercise.)

Visualization exercise:

> Close your eyes in a quiet, comfortable place. After a few cleansing breaths, imagine yourself as a toddler. See how round you are as you roll on the floor or pull yourself up to stand. Hear the adults saying, "What a darling child." Feel happiness in knowing that they are talking about you. The fat on the child is okay, because it is natural for all children to have baby fat. Then, picture yourself as a young teenager, just starting to mature. Your body needs to grow at this time; it needs some extra fat, too. Now, see yourself moving into adulthood. Your body is not the same. Finally, imagine yourself at 90-years-old. What would you look like? Bodies change. Relax. Get comfortable with this idea. Appreciate what nature gave you.

When I look back at pictures of myself with anorexia, I look so thin. I can't believe that I thought I was fat. Now I know that I wasn't thinking clearly and I was overly hard on myself.

It took a long time for me to get used to my maintenance weight. I was depressed until I realized that being thin hadn't changed my life at all. Matter of fact, it was a lot better at a healthier weight.

Relaxation

While our culture embraces a hard-work ethic and rewards people for being productive, being too busy can have serious negative consequences. This is the case for individuals suffering with anorexia whose minds are constantly racing and whose bodies are pushed to the limits of endurance.

In addition to putting tremendous stress on the body, constant activity is a way to avoid problems or issues that need attention. In fact, keeping busy can become an addiction if it distracts us from painful emotions or memories. Many anorexics say that they feel like they *have* to keep busy or they will be overwhelmed by their feelings.

The most negative consequence of overactivity is that it disconnects you from your inner self and tricks you into thinking that you are only as good as your accomplishments. You then become a "human doing" instead of a "human being." Your life, which is on constant overload, lacks meaning, because you don't slow down enough to feel connected to it.

Taking rest and relaxation might sound easy, but it can be quite difficult. Even as you are sitting quietly, your mind can still be moving at breakneck speed. Fears, worries, and painful feelings can come up and cause tremendous inner turmoil. For this reason, experiment with exercises to both quiet your mind and relax your body; and, keep your journal handy for insights, explorations, and companionship.

Practice your relaxation techniques on a regular basis, beginning with even as little as a few minutes a day. Remind yourself that you are worth this precious practice and that, over time, the benefits will continue to grow. Quiet the voice in your mind that tells you that you should be doing something else, and turn your awareness inward. Free from frenetic activity, your body will be able to use its energy to heal itself and reduce tension and stress. You will be better able to hear the voice in your heart.

There are many books on relaxation, and we suggest browsing your local bookstore and library. Here is a list of suggested ways to relax:

RELAXATION TECHNIQUES

- Meditate
- Create opportunities to laugh
- Take a walk
- Do deep breathing exercises
- Practice yoga or T'ai Chi
- Stretch
- Pray
- Listen to soothing music
- Get a massage
- Sit quietly in candlelight
- Take a bath
- Nap
- Sit in a beautiful or holy place
- Watch your fish, pet your cat, walk the dog

Relaxation exercise:

Give yourself at least a 15 or 20 minute slot of time. Comfortably sit or lie down in a peaceful spot. Gently close your eyes, and remind yourself that you are a good person, deserving of great love and respect. Silently count to six as you inhale, again to six as you hold your breath, and once more as you exhale. Repeat this three times to slow down and focus your mind. Then repeat "I am," with each breath. (You may substitute other words, prayers, or a mantra, for "I am," but it is helpful to maintain repetition.) Try not to be occupied by your thoughts, but allow them to pass through your mind and bring your repetition back in focus. If you have a problem or question in the forefront of your mind, make note and then go back to repetition. This takes practice, and there will be times when your mind will refuse to slow down, but eventually you will be able to enjoy a state of deep relaxation.

When I first began to eat, I would panic, so I lay on my bed, followed my breathing and made myself think of good things. This calmed me down.

In the beginning, I meditated twice every day for 20 minutes before breakfast and dinner. This made eating easier because I was more in touch with the inner "me" who wanted to get well.

My mind goes a million miles a minute. I have a hot tub in a cedar room, with plants, where I go when I feel the most stressed. I light some candles and can feel calm.

Strengthen Your Boundaries

Like the invisible line between two countries, your boundary is a border that separates you from others. It helps define you as a person with unique feelings, opinions, experiences, and values. Physical boundaries enable you to control the kind and amount of contact you have with other people, like whether or not you want to be hugged or how close you stand in a conversation. Emotional boundaries protect your feelings, such as when you choose to limit your contact with someone who says hurtful or thoughtless things.

Strong boundaries keep you safe by setting appropriate guidelines for your relationships with people or situations. They help you choose what to let into your experience and what to keep out. They are a sign that you know who you are and how you want to be treated. Strong boundaries assert that you are a person worth protecting—that you matter.

Weak boundaries, on the other hand, are a sign that you *don't* think you worth protecting—that you *don't* matter. There are many reasons why you might feel this way. Your feelings might have been consistently invalidated or ignored. You may have endured emotional or physical abuse, or been treated with a general lack of respect. Other people might have taken control over your decisions, making you feel powerless and unimportant. Whatever the reason, weak boundaries mean that you don't have a strong sense of yourself as separate from other people; you are more likely to do what pleases them than what pleases you.

Under these circumstances, anorexia serves as a form of boundary. It asserts your right to live your own life in your own way, and forces people to recognize you as an independent, separate person. An emaciated body is a powerful message that you are in charge and well-protected. It is an impenetrable wall that keeps others out, providing a haven of sorts that no one can take away. However, the boundaries that you set with anorexia are not satisfying or fulfilling, because they are based on your feeling powerless and unimportant.

One goal of recovery is to strengthen your healthy boundaries. This becomes more possible by recognizing your own worth and using your voice. Use "I messages," clearly stating what the other person is doing, how that makes you feel, and what you would like to be different. For example, "When you tell me you know what is best for me, I feel stupid. I'd like you to hear what I think is best for me."

Treat yourself with love and respect, and in that way show other people how you want to be treated. Remind yourself that you are entitled to your feelings and desires. You have a right to be safe. You are a worthwhile, important person with unique gifts to give. You matter.

I moved away from my father and limited the phone calls. That gave me more freedom to have my own voice, instead of listening to him and doing what he wanted.

Learning to say "no" was hard for me because I didn't want to disappoint anyone. I always thought about the other person instead of myself. Now I know that if I say "yes" when I don't mean it, I feel terrible about myself later.

Cultivate Healthy Relationships

Anorexia is often born in bad relationships. Abuse, harassment, feelings of invisibility or powerlessness, a lack of love or emotional support are all legitimate reasons why a person might want to distance themselves with an eating disorder. Anorexia appears to be a safe, simple relationship taking the place of the more complicated, confusing real-life ones. Unfortunately, though, it can provide none of the feelings of connection, authenticity, respect, and sheer joy of a healthy relationship.

You have spent so much energy on your relationship with anorexia that you may have forgotten how, in fact, a relationship with a person works. Maybe you think other people expect you to be an independent person, self-sufficient, with few needs or problems, and this is what you have done by becoming anorexic. But the challenge of recovery is not for you to be independent of people, but rather that you maintain your independence *while in relationships with others*. Maintaining a sense of yourself while in relationships is a lot different from not being in a relationship at all.

Just as you are getting to know yourself, let others know who you are. Learn to share your true self—your feelings, hopes, fears and dreams. Talk about more than just your anorexia and related fears. Discuss a variety of topics. In this way, you will create for yourself a network of friends, family members, and professionals to travel with you on your path.

Rediscovering friendship and intimacy without your illness requires courage and practice. Sharing your inner self with others can be very difficult if you have been hurt in the past, or if you are afraid of what other people might think of you if they knew the seriousness of your problem. Here is another recovery area in which to shower yourself with compassion. As you gradually get to know and like yourself, you will have more confidence to share. The bottom line is, you have committed to being anorexia-free, to living a life filled with honest, authentic relationships. And you will get there. You will.

Recovery is not an overnight process. People around you, even those who love you the most, may become impatient and make comments that cause you to feel ashamed or embarrassed. You may find yourself feeling guilty for not healing as fast as they would like. Your healing process, however, is yours, and you are entitled to complete it as you see fit, in your own, unique way, no matter what it looks like to anybody else.

Try these seemingly simple ideas to kick-start your way to new relationships:

MAKING NEW RELATIONSHIPS

- Be honest at all times.
- Write a letter or email to a friend.
- Volunteer in a retirement home; "adopt" one of the residents.
- Baby-sit or play with a pet; kids and animals love unconditionally!
- "Role play" conversations with a therapist or in the privacy of your room with an empty chair.
- Take a class.
- Join a club or organization.
- Go to the park and people-watch. Imagine yourself making friends. Most people are shy, so why not take the initiative and say "hello" first?

Remember that anorexia is a selfish companion that isolates you and keeps others at a distance. Befriend people and invite them into your life to replace the anorexia. Let them in to support you, know you, and celebrate with you. You deserve life-affirming connections and healthy relationships.

When I finally began to emerge from my anorexic shell after 12 years, I discovered that I am a person who loves other people! I now have several close friends and feel lucky.

Sharing my recovery with others helped me see that I'm a worthy person. I am good enough just being me.

After a few months of recovery work, my relationship with my parents began to improve. Now, we are closer than ever.

Spiritual Pursuits

People with anorexia have stopped growing, not only physically and emotionally, but spiritually, as well. They often lack a sense of meaning in their lives and feel disconnected from others. Even though they have accomplished something few can—significant weight loss—they are plagued by negativity and an overall low opinion of themselves. Many feel undeserving of food, symbolic of their alienation from life itself.

A powerful tool for transforming these feelings is what we call "spiritual pursuits," or recognizing the spirit that dwells within ourselves and everyone, apart from our minds and bodies. For most people, this also means connecting with a greater sense of spirit, which is called many names, such as: God, Higher Power, the Self, collective unconscious, etc. In fact, many recovered anorexics and bulimics have said that their recoveries were inspired by a glimmer of this inner spirit urging them to get better.

The truth is that each of us has a source of love within ourselves. The experience of this inner light can give us feelings of being connected with our spiritual self and with other people, and provide us with guidance and strength to make changes. Looking within can put us in touch with our capacity for compassion, creativity, humor, and kindness. It can give us an appreciation for our bodies as the vehicle for our self-discovery. Ultimately, recognizing our inherent self-worth can transform our lives forever.

Trying to describe this inner source to someone who may not believe such a thing exists is like describing a hot fudge sundae to a person who does not eat. Its existence must be experienced, not just believed on an intellectual level. Experiment with different activities to help you to be more spiritually aware, such as: meditation, prayer, spiritual readings, visualization, yoga, paying attention to your breathing, and relaxation exercises. Quiet your mind and hush the negative self-talk. Listen to the voice in your heart without directing your thoughts. Spend time devoted to reaching this inner source, and in so doing, affirm that you are important and that your inner life has value.

As the awareness of your inner love grows, you will also begin to experience the world as a reflection of that love. You will recognize this greatness in others, even if they themselves are unaware of its existence. You will see that everyone has issues in their lives, just as you do, and be able to treat them and yourself with compassion. You will discover other activities which make you feel equally uplifted, like volunteer work, gardening, art, music, inspirational writing, being in nature, and, for someone in recovery from an eating disorder, even cooking! Remember, just as your body yearns to be fed, so does your spirit.

Spirituality is a common theme in self-help literature, particularly by authors who have overcome problems with food. Here are a few insights:

To heal yourself from your eating problem, you need to integrate your inner or spiritual self into your daily life. . . . The healing process exists within you, but it also extends beyond you because it is part of a greater benevolent force. Consequently, you don't need to make healing happen in your own limited ways. Instead, you need to create the right conditions so that it can unfold in your life. Healing happens by itself when you open up to it.

Viola Fodor, Desperately Seeking Self

Healing requires a willingness on our part to give up. . . the illu-sion that when we are thin we will be happy. . . Moving steadfastly inward to the center of our Self, we can discover a truly rich and fulfilling life.

Jane E. Latimer, BEYOND THE FOOD GAME

You can make the most of any journey by staying alert to the God-force in your life. . . I encourage you to include God more fully in your struggles with weight.

Laura Rose, LIFE ISN'T WEIGHED ON THE BATHROOM SCALE

Some use religion as the starting point for developing positive self-esteem: If God created you and loves you regardless of your weak-nesses and mistakes, then you are always worthy and valuable in an absolute and unconditional way. You do not have to believe in God, however, to develop unconditional self-acceptance. . . You can choose unconditional self-acceptance instead of all the mea-suring, comparing, and judging you have been taught to do.

Susan Kano, MAKING PEACE WITH FOOD

When we practice love, we are making a connection with our real selves. This love cuts through the layers of false selves that we wear for protection, and makes clear that we are at our core, not flawed, but divine.

Lindsey Hall & Leigh Cohn, SELF-ESTEEM TOOLS FOR RECOVERY

Let Go

Control is a complicated subject when discussing anorexia, because it is somewhat of a paradox. Do you feel that you are in control of food and weight, or that anorexia nervosa controls you?

Some anorexics rigidly control their food intake because they are unable to control other areas of their lives, such as leaving home or a divorce in the family, but no situation was ever made better by not eating. Also, although losing weight in a culture that glorifies thinness can provide feelings of competence and pride, these feelings are based on underlying low self-esteem and insecurity. Finally, while there is a certain sense of safety in doing things in a predictable manner, for instance eating exactly the same way every meal or weighing yourself at the same time every day, these rigid behaviors are a prison.

And so the paradox is this: although it might appear to the outside observer that you are extremely controlling, in fact, your illness is controlling you. You have no choice—you believe that to feel good about yourself, you have to keep losing weight. You have let anorexia make your choices for you.

Perfectionism is a form of control, with the same effects. Being the best or being perfect at something, whether it be weight loss or having a superclean house, provides feelings of accomplishment, worth, and success. It can also be a way of avoiding other problems. However, perfectionism is both a dangerous pursuit and a heavy burden. If you are a perfectionist, what you do in the present is never good enough because you think you could do better in the future. Your flaws are magnified. You constantly compete with yourself and others. Always on the lookout for external standards, you judge yourself unmercifully for not meeting them. There is always a better grade, a better performance, or another pound to lose. Pursuing perfection has no end or reward.

To recover from anorexia, you have to let go. Recognize that control, for you or for anyone, is an illusion. Real control, or a *real* sense of personal power, comes from listening and being guided by the voice in your heart. Doing everything perfectly will not necessarily make you happier, healthier, or a better person. Take risks. Give yourself permission to make mistakes, and by the same token, you will have more compassion for others. Trust your body's natural wisdom. Susan Kano, a recovered anorexic, wrote about trusting your body in an essay, "Leap of Faith" in the book *Full Lives:*

> I call the decision to eat spontaneously a "leap of faith" because the body's wisdom is not something one can touch, see, or quantify. I had to have faith that my body would regulate my appetite and weight, but there were no guarantees it would work . . . Hence, I embarked on spontaneous eating with intense doubt, anxiety, and fear, and it took a leap of faith to proceed despite those feelings (p. 111) . . . This is what the leap of faith is all about: recognizing the difference between things you should control with your intellect versus things best left to your body's wisdom. You relinquish control of your appetite and weight to a different part of yourself and thereby draw strength and support from an inner realm (p. 121).

The Serenity Prayer, which is recited at Overeaters Anonymous and other 12-step meetings, may have deep meaning for you: "God give me the serenity to accept the things I can't change, the courage to change the things I can, and the wisdom to know the difference." Think about it. You do have a choice.

I always thought I had to do everything just so. Becoming more relaxed about my perfectionism was difficult but liberating.

I was afraid that if I started eating I wouldn't be able to stop. I thought my appetite was so huge that I had to control it. I found out that wasn't true. Now, I eat normally and stop when I feel full.

I didn't want to be controlled, I wanted to be in control. Not eating help me to do that. But life just happens, nobody is in control of anything. Once I accepted that, I was able to start eating.

Express Yourself

Anorexics have difficulty expressing their feelings and needs. With the same rigidity that they deny physical hunger by not eating, they refuse to acknowledge emotional cravings as well. Hiding feelings and needs is safer than revealing them.

Some anorexics fear that if they do begin to express themselves, they will let loose feelings which they think are unacceptable or dangerous, such as anger or disappointment. They hold back in relationships for fear of rejection, or to avoid conflict or confrontation. Women especially are timid about their needs, as though it is unladylike to be assertive, opinionated, loud, sexual, or to have large appetites of any kind.

Many anorexics fear recovery, because they (perhaps subconsciously) think if they allow their weight and behaviors to normalize, they will lose their means of expression. They wonder who will care about them, how will their needs get met, how will they be heard, are they worthy of support? Remaining with the *status quo* is easier, and less scary.

However, you do not have to let anorexia speak for you. You can learn to say everything that anorexia currently communicates for you in healthier ways. Finding and using your voice means you are taking care of yourself. Being assertive is difficult when you are questioning your own worth, but your recovery depends on it. If saying, "I need," feels uncomfortable, try saying instead, "My heart needs me to..." or "My heart is telling me to talk about..."

Also, if you have a hard time getting the words out, consider other means of expressing yourself such as through art or music, dancing, or writing poetry. If you have something difficult to say to someone, write it in a letter first, giving yourself the option of sending it or not. Remember, you are a unique individual with unique needs, abilities, and things to offer. Express yourself and be heard.

I had to figure out exactly what I needed and ask for it. It sounds simple, but I think saying the words out loud is one of the hardest things I've ever done.

I'm a shy person by nature, so speaking up was tough. I felt like, "Who am I to be asking for anything?" Somewhere along the way I began to understand that I wasn't being demanding at all, just honest.

My eating disorder gave me the autonomy I needed. Even though I wasn't talking, people were listening to what my behavior was saying. The trick in recovery was learning to use my voice and healthy behaviors to make people listen and respect me as an individual.

Focus on Recovery

This chapter has given you many ideas to think about, as well as suggestions for activities to help you in your recovery from anorexia. But ideas and suggestions are not enough. At some point, you have to put them into practice. Thinking about recovery is a lot different that the experience of it.

For this reason, it is important that you set up a schedule in order to incorporate recovery activities into your daily life. We have discussed the benefits of writing in a journal. Why not set aside time every day or two specifically for your journal? We have stressed taking time to relax, thinking more positive thoughts, and trying new things. Why not schedule a meditation of some kind every morning, repeat an affirmation every day, or explore a new activity once a week?

Taking into account where you are in your recovery process and the kinds of things you most enjoy, come up with a schedule of activities. The idea is not how much you do, but rather that you focus on recovery in some way every day. Use a calendar if it will help you stay on track. By devoting time to positive, enriching experiences and getting to know who you are apart from the anorexia, you will experience moments of wellness and clarity. These moments will build on each other to help you live a healthier and happier life.

CHAPTER 6

Healthy Eating and Healthy Weight

In addition to working on the issues that underlie your eating disorder, you also have to work on the more practical matters of eating and reaching a healthy target weight. This work is extremely challenging, demanding that you sometimes do things you would prefer not to do. You must sit with physical discomfort and fear, and stay focused on the goal of your overall health and well being, even during times when you feel like giving up. It also demands that you let go of the one thing that has identified you for so long—your excessive thinness.

You might think that your fears about food and eating will dissipate on their own once the underlying issues have been resolved, but this is rarely the case. You might have been told that your eating disorder isn't about food, and that therefore you should not address food issues. But you are faced with food and weight fears daily, and you need a plan to handle them.

There most certainly will be times when the choice to eat is extremely difficult, but there are things that you can do to get through them successfully. Affirm that there is a healthy weight for you which you want to reach. Get in touch with the part of you that recognizes the importance of eating—no one else can do that for you. Use the techniques that we discussed in the last chapter, such as journal writing, relaxation, and talking with others to make the process easier. Make a list of the pros and cons of weight gain to convince yourself that you are on the right track. Do whatever works for you.

Set Point and Metabolism

You need to understand the concept of "set point." This means that everyone's body has a particular weight range that it fights to maintain, which is primarily determined by heredity, age, health, and activity level. In other words, our bodies *want* to be a certain weight—the one nature gave us—because it is the most efficient and healthy for our particular body. When a small amount of food is eaten, our metabolism slows down in order to benefit from every calorie. When a large amount is eaten, it speeds up to fully digest. In this way, our bodies work naturally to keep us at our healthiest weight.

Chances are your metabolism is considerably slower than normal because you have been restricting your food intake for so long. Essentially, the body has interpreted this as "starvation" and has slowed down to preserve its stored energy. When you begin to eat more normally, your metabolism will speed up, making it possible for you to eat without gaining more weight than is right for your body.

Think about a weight range of between five and ten pounds that you feel is a reachable goal. Look at your family for clues. Ask your nutritionist or dietician for their estimation of what would be an appropriate target weight based on your age, height, body type and gender. Mentally prepare yourself to return to a "generally healthy" size, and visualize what that will look like. Affirm that restoring your body weight is a priority for your recovery and that you are willing to do whatever it takes. Your body is an efficient, intelligent wonder; trust it by working towards your set point.

Healthy Eating: Where to Begin

Relearning how to eat in a normal way is extremely frightening for someone who is used to eating only in prescribed amounts. You may be unfamiliar with signals of hunger and fullness, which regulate what and how much to eat. Relying on your instincts may result in your continuing to eat less than your body needs or only foods that you consider "safe."

Meal Planning

For this reason, we suggest that you seek the professional help of a nutritionist or dietician who is familiar with both anorexia and its treatment. By taking into consideration your food preferences and life-style, they can help design a balanced eating plan that is comfortable for you. They can ensure that you are getting all of the essential nutrients that your body needs, while pacing your weight gain to minimize your panic. They can also support you emotionally when you face the food fears that every anorexic encounters in the course of normalizing his or her eating.

If professional help is not available, create your own meal plan. Design it on paper. Include what foods you are going to eat, in what proportion, and at what time. This will help you eat even when you don't feel like eating—which might have more to do with your perceptions and fears than your body's actual needs. Start with foods with which you feel safe, then slowly introduce new foods as you gain confidence. Make an effort to stick to this plan, returning to it even if you stray for one meal.

Timing of Meals

Most experts recommend eating three meals a day, with a balance of protein, carbohydrate and fat at each one, as well as two or three between-meal snacks. However, you might feel more comfortable with six small meals, or eating every couple of hours. Due to delayed gastric emptying, a side-effect of anorexia which causes feelings of fullness, most people find it more tolerable to eat small meals throughout the day. There's nothing wrong with eating at set intervals until you are able to recognize and respond to your body's internal cues.

Portion Size

One challenge is to be able to eat "normal" portions, which you can find in a good nutrition book or on food packaging labels. It is helpful to know, for example, that three to four ounces of meat equals one portion, and that beans are measured by the half cup per serving, as is cooked rice and cottage cheese. Learning portion size helps you feel in control by assuring that you are not eating too much. Some recovering anorexics cannot tolerate eating even normal portions in the beginning. Although a day's calorie intake may initially be low, refeeding can begin with smaller sizes, starting with ice-cube size portions, if necessary, eaten every two to three hours, rather than starting with full meals.

Which Foods?

Certainly, an indicator of a strong recovery is the ability to eat a wide variety of foods in normal portions without undue stress.

But this is a goal that is usually reached after a great many trials and over a long period of time, sometimes years.

If you have been a severe restrictor, consider starting out with a variety of easily-digestible foods, such as egg whites for protein, white rice, and canned or fresh pears. Depending on how the body responds, you can rebuild from there. Other generally bland foods to be slowly introduced include: fish, turkey, chicken, and juiced or pureed fruits and vegetables. Reintroducing the body to food is almost like going on a baby-food diet.

Also, in the early stages, some experts recommend increasing the amount of high-quality protein consumed, such as: fish, poultry, eggs, legumes, dairy, and tofu. Additional protein will cause an increase in energy quickly and does not lead to major weight gain due to water retention. This will give you feelings of confidence and more trust in your body. Since protein takes longer to digest, you may feel full long after you have eaten, giving you the opportunity to recognize hunger when it does return. A vitamin/mineral supplement will help to ensure proper nutrition.

Eventually, you will be able to extend beyond the foods which you now consider "safe." Proceed at your own pace so that you are not scared back into restricting behaviors. Restoring weight is a delicate balance between increasing the amounts or frequency of your meals while challenging yourself to take risks. Identify your goals in this area and strive to reach them. Perhaps try a new food every week, or promise yourself one delicious dessert every day, week, or month. Rely on your support team for reassurance, such as using an "eating buddy" to sit with you during meals.

Special Situations

Eating at restaurants, going to parties, and attending gatherings are particularly anxiety-provoking for anorexics. Often, menus are elaborate, and gatherings are food-centered. Additionally, many restaurants serve portions that are too large for most people. Thus, it is important not only to get to know what a healthy portion size looks like, but to recognize when you may need to use a relaxation technique to help get you through a party or meal away from home.

If you are served more food than you want, you can separate appropriate portion sizes and put the rest of your serving into a take-home container before or after the meal has ended. Another option is to order from the appetizer menu, or share a meal with a friend. If you are invited for dinner and are served something you feel uncomfortable about, don't panic. Take a deep breath and try to relax. If necessary, briefly explain to your host that you are following a meal plan that is helping you to overcome an eating disorder. It does not mean you are relapsing if you simply cannot eat what is served. Eat what you can, and if that was not enough, eat more when you get home.

Any fears and reactions that arise are okay. You can't expect to become a stress-free party-goer overnight. Remind yourself that you chose to stop the self-destructive behaviors of anorexia in order to live a more happy and healthy life. Part of this involves reacquainting yourself with the social aspect of eating. Challenging yourself by making and accepting invitations out is a recovery task that can help free you from anorexia.

Getting Past Food Fears

Confronting food fears is an important part of recovering from an eating disorder, but actually doing this is far from easy. Most anorexics have a limited list of what they will allow themselves to eat. Expanding that list is a challenge every recovering anorexic must face; it is part of the process.

In many cases, food fears are perpetuated by false beliefs about food and weight. For instance, the idea that eating sugar in any form will cause weight gain is not true. Equally false is the belief that eating only fruits and vegetables is a healthy vegetarian diet. (Reiff & Reiff 1992, p.145) While these distortions might help preserve a sense of safety and identity, they stand in the way of recovery and must be challenged.

Some recovering anorexics say that they are more able to eat a previously forbidden food if they exchange it for one of their "safe" foods. Others find that buying and eating single serving meals, with caloric content clearly marked, allows them to eat with less fear. Still others have been able to begin eating because their loved ones wanted them to, eventually eating because *they* wanted to. Whatever system you choose to use, the goal is to increase the variety and amount of food you eat, with growing confidence.

One method for desensitizing yourself from your fear of particular foods is to begin by choosing one forbidden food that you would like to eat. Then, "just do it." Eat that food, concentrating on its texture and flavor. Troublesome thoughts will crash in on you as you are doing this, but persistently push them away. Consciously refocus your attention back to enjoying the flavor. Once you are finished, set a timer for ten minutes and then allow yourself to think about all the usual "remedies" you had for eating a forbidden food (like starving, exercising, etc.), but do not engage in any of them! After ten minutes, when the timer goes off, firmly say out loud, "It's only food! Who cares? I deserve to eat without fear!" Then force yourself to do something else. Perhaps write in your journal, call a friend, or go to a park. When the worries about that particular food creep back in, as they inevitably will, redirect your thoughts to the new task at hand and affirm to yourself, calmly and simply that you are okay. Remind yourself that every food is fine in moderation and a normal serving of any food will not cause you to become obese.

It is also helpful to ask yourself, "Is my concern over this particular food filling space to avoid some other thought or feeling?" You might be able to pinpoint a circumstance or set of feelings that are troubling you. Whether or not this is the case, asking yourself this question and exploring it as a possibility circumvents your negative thought patterns around the food you have just eaten—and that is one of your goals.

Be patient with yourself. It takes time to change long-term behaviors and reactions. But it is possible and you can do it.

Physical Complications

Although restoring body weight can provoke overwhelming anxiety for someone with an eating disorder, learning how your body will change helps. Armed with some basic biological facts, a willingness to ask questions, and a commitment to support yourself with regular self-talk, the process of healing your body can be less mysterious and frightening.

Edema, or fluid retention, for example, is a condition which occurs when restricting, vomiting, laxative or diuretic abuse are stopped. The body holds onto water, which causes your weight to go up. This is a fairly normal consequence of refeeding in the early stages. In addition, body protein is destroyed by starvation. As you restore your weight to non-starvation level, new proteins are created through a process called tissue synthesis, potentially causing weight gain. Your physician can explain to you that both of these conditions are temporary and are the result of your body returning to a normal, balanced state.

Another side-effect of starvation is slow gastric emptying, meaning that food is slow to leave your stomach. It takes time for the body to readjust to normal food intake. During the first few months of recovery, you may feel bloated even after eating a small amount of food. Another possibility might be that you are experiencing an allergy or an intolerance to dairy or gluten, which also contributes to bloating. Ask your doctor.

As you approach your target weight, you may be tempted to return to or increase your exercise regime, not only to purge unwanted calories, but to alleviate your anxiety. Try not to. Consider stabilizing at an intermediary weight for a while, and then return to your efforts. Remember, the only way to recover is through this process. Stick with it no matter how long it takes. Be patient; your anorexia didn't develop overnight, and its effects won't disappear instantly. Gently remind yourself that you are "restoring" the weight that your body needs in order for you to be healthy and strong.

Emotional Issues

Underlying your inability to eat are sensitive emotional issues, which will undoubtedly surface as your body begins to change. If anorexia has provided you with a sense of protection, gaining weight will seem to threaten your safety. If you have used your anorexia to speak for you, you may feel silenced. If being thin has given you a sense of achievement and competence, you may fear that you will never be as good at anything else. You might even discover that you don't feel deserving of food or deserving of a happy life.

While these issues are extremely painful, they are, in actuality, pointing you toward recovery. Whatever it is that keeps you from eating is exactly what you need to explore. If you need protection, try assertiveness training, stress management, or self-defense classes. For a means of expression, use your voice, writing, or art. Work on becoming good at something other than starvation.

Watching my body change filled me with panic. I kept thinking my thighs and legs were huge, and I would freak out. Finally, I started forcing myself to just not look at them. I knew what my goal weight was and I knew I wasn't there yet, so I kept reminding myself of that. I listened to a lot of relaxation tapes, too. That definitely helped me to calm down.

I had a big problem with edema. My whole body swelled. It was like my worst nightmare had come true. My doctor and nutritionist were really great, though. They reassured me that it would go away soon. They encouraged me to get myself involved in activities that would take my mind off of it. I had a really hard time riding it out, but I'm glad I did.

I forced myself to take risks. It was always important to me to be able to someday eat like a normal person who doesn't have an eating disorder. I wanted to be able to eat whatever I wanted, wherever I wanted, without driving myself or the people I was with crazy.

Seeing that I could eat something I was afraid of and not get fat overnight or die from it helped me tremendously.

Everyone always says it's not about the food, but you know what? Some of it is! It may not be the root, but it is definitely a branch that you have to recognize and address if you want to get better.

CHAPTER **7**

How to
Stay Committed

Recovery is a long journey marked with steep hills, deep valleys, and an occasional flat plain. Although you can usually recognize headway when you look back over weeks and months of effort, the daily work of recovery can be hard and discouraging. Sometimes it may seem that you aren't making any progress at all. You might be plagued by feelings of ambivalence, slips and setbacks, or a slide into full-blown relapse. When this happens, you will surely wonder how to pick yourself up and move ahead.

Perhaps knowing that you will encounter these obstacles will lessen their power over you. Read books, such as this one, which can give you some idea of what to expect along your path to wellness. Talk to other people who have overcome eating disorders, and ask them how they stayed motivated. Brainstorm in your journal all the reasons why your life will be better once you do recover, and read that list often. Talk with your therapist. Do whatever you can think of to remind yourself that no matter how long and difficult your journey may seem to you at times, you will not give up.

Ambivalence

Ambivalence is a particularly difficult obstacle to overcome because it drains you of motivation. Ambivalence raises questions. Why work hard if you are not even sure you want to get better? What can you do when recovery feels so much harder than remaining where you are?

First, ambivalent feelings are a completely normal part of recovery. As we have said, anorexia has been taking care of you in many ways, and the prospect of letting it go may feel as though you are heading into battle without your weapons. Of course, you might not feel like going forward! But even though remaining anorexic might be more familiar and more comfortable, it has taken control of your life. Fight your feelings of ambivalence with courage and determination, and take your life back.

Second, your conflicting feelings have no bearing on your ability to free yourself. It is possible to go ahead and make steps towards recovery even when you don't want to. Go ahead and try a new food even though the thought terrifies you. Talk about your feelings even though you are embarrassed. In overcoming your fear and resistance, you will be rewarded with feelings of accomplishment and pride. You are in charge of your anorexia, and not vice versa.

When your motivation wanes, remind yourself that this is normal, but don't let your guard down. Interpret your ambivalence as a signal that you need to make time to check in with yourself. Are you tired, afraid, frustrated? Ask your support team for encouragement. Ask your inner self for the strength to persevere. You are worth fighting for.

When I went to my first therapy appointment, 50% of me wanted to get better, but 50% did not! How could I give up something that was such a fundamental part of my life? Who would I be without anorexia? Slowly I began to realize that I was a person who was worth fighting for and that other people would like me even if I wasn't anorexic.

What it all comes down to is this: Do I want these eating disorders to destroy me, or do I want to keep fighting and hopefully win? The answer isn't always easy.

I want a new life. I know that in recovery, I will encounter many times of weakness, and can only hope for the strength to fight at those times. I know in my heart and soul that I want to give this every ounce of strength that I have.

If you can't think of a reason to recover, just remember the little things in life, like the smell of fresh cut grass, butterflies, wild flowers growing on a hillside. These things are waiting for you.

Slips and Setbacks

Nearly everyone backslides at some point on their journey. Although this is more likely to happen early in the process, a slip or setback can occur at any time. The trick is not to berate yourself for having them. Remember that there is no such thing as a perfect recovery; there is just doing your best at any given time with the experience you have. You are learning how to live in a completely new way, and slips and setbacks can be excellent teachers.

Instead of putting yourself down for skipping a meal, take the time to look at *why* you were unable to eat. Instead of beating yourself up for overexercising, try to understand what was happening at the time. Can you pinpoint possible triggers? Have you been upset about something that feels difficult to face? Did you need something but weren't sure how to ask for it? Did you need a break from your feelings?

Once you understand what triggered your slip, think about other things to do next time that are not self-destructive. Call someone for support. Read or write in your journal. Leave the house and go for a walk. Respond in a more nurturing, self-loving way.

Slips and setbacks are opportunities to learn more about your anorexia and what it represents. Understand and learn from these teachers, and then move on.

I had a lot of slips in the beginning. As I got further into recovery, they lessened to the point of nonexistence.

The last time I fell back into my old behaviors, it felt like a roller coaster that wouldn't want to stop. The best thing I did was to go back to my support group. They assured me that I wasn't a disappointment and put me back on track.

I have to say that, in spite of pain and depression, there is a little voice inside of me that whispers, "Rise again and go on!"

Relapse

Relapse, or returning to anorexic ways, occurs for some people. Usually stress pushes the person to revert to old, familiar coping mechanisms in spite of the progress that has already been made. Regardless of the cause, it is important that you familiarize yourself with the warning signs.

RELAPSE WARNING SIGNS

- Increased preoccupation with food and weight
- Skipping meals
- Desire to be isolated
- An increased focus on calories and fat content
- Frequently weighing
- Inability to talk honestly with support network
- Overexercising
- Feeling guilty after eating
- Planning ways to compensate for eating (i.e. eating less at the next meal)
- Feeling hopeless and depressed
- Self-destructive thoughts
- Negative self-talk

If you notice any of these signs, talk to your therapist or a support person. Let them into your world by describing what is *really* going on. Be completely honest. It's okay to ask for help; it's okay to lean on someone. When you feel a relapse coming on, you need to regain perspective, and talking about it gently lets the air out of that about-to-burst relapse bubble.

Immediately set aside time to examine what is going on in your life. Try to sit quietly and ask yourself what is causing you to feel as if you need anorexia to survive. Write in your journal. Notice how your body feels. Take a deep breath and remind yourself that all your feelings are okay and manageable. Then acknowledge yourself for even stopping to face your problems. In simply recognizing that something is brewing and needs your attention, you are practicing self-love and are farther along the recovery path then ever.

If you do find yourself caught in a full-blown relapse; don't give up. It means that your work is not finished, but hope is by no means lost. Remind yourself that in committing to letting go of anorexia, you have acknowledged that you want to be able to handle life, with its full spectrum of ups and downs. Working through a relapse will teach you more about treating yourself with compassion, forgiveness, and acceptance—things that will assist you for the rest of your life. Pretty soon, friends and acquaintances will be coming to you for advice!

I was devastated to find myself in relapse after spending half a year feeling recovered. Looking back, I can see that I just couldn't handle my chaotic life, and my coping skills still felt so new that they didn't carry me through. I had to work with renewed effort to get back on track.

I had one year of recovery and then a horrible relapse. I was really stressed out, and to be honest, I saw all of the warning signs and ignored them. I think if I'd done something about it when I first noticed, I probably would have been okay. The positive side of it is that although it took me six more months of hard work, I recovered from my relapse and I've been fine for several years. I'm confident that I won't have another one, because when I see signs approaching, I'll talk about the problem right away and head it off.

Holding onto Hope

Although there are times when holding onto hope seems like the hardest thing in the world, doing so is crucial. What is hope anyway? Hope is believing there is light even when you can't see it. Hope is holding on to the belief that your life will get better even when you have no idea how that could be possible. It means having faith in yourself even when you feel the most down.

You may not believe it, but most people think poorly of themselves. It is a rare person who thinks, "Yes, I really live up to my highest potential all the time. I always make the right decisions. I am a great person." Most people have a hard time liking themselves, much less loving themselves! But the truth is that everyone has an inner source of love and strength—they just don't know it. Most people don't take the time to get to know who they are, and have no idea that they possess such qualities.

This, then, is the greatest reward of recovery, and the primary reason to hold onto hope: Facing and overcoming anorexia is a means for gaining true self-love, which then affects your whole life in positive ways—the people you meet, the situations you are in, and the decisions you have to make. When you know how to love yourself, your life is forever changed.

Right now, imagine that you are a great person—kind, generous, creative, funny, light. How does that feel? It is surely more pleasant than thinking the worst of yourself! There really is light inside of you. You are a great person—you just don't believe it. Your task is to remove all of the obstacles in your path, anorexia as well as any others, that prevent you from letting this light shine.

To remind yourself that you have not lost your hope, recognize that you picked up this book! Each appointment you keep to see your therapist, doctor, or nutritionist is also evidence that your optimism has not vanished. You are showing up for your treatment; you are reading and searching for answers. All of this proves that somewhere inside yourself exists the light of hope.

Healing from anorexia is about embracing yourself instead of pushing yourself away. It is about accepting, with gentleness, all of the difficulties you have suffered, and learning from them. Recovery is about experiencing your feelings, as raw and scary as they sometimes feel. When you come to a place where you choose to know and love yourself through these struggles, you are living the definition of hope.

Having hope for recovery is what makes recovery possible. I once worked with a clinician who told me, "Once you have an eating disorder, you always have an eating disorder," and I found that to be one of the most depressing things I had ever heard. I finally found other clinicians who believed in me, and that has made all the difference in the world.

Sometimes it's difficult to have hope. It feels like you're working so hard and getting nowhere. This is when you have to stop and take careful inventory of your progress. It's important to see how far you have come and not how far you have left to go.

CHAPTER 8

A Guide for
Parents and Loved Ones

When we see people we love in pain, our natural reaction is to want to relieve that pain. Even though we cannot do this for someone who is suffering with an eating disorder, there are ways to help them. Anorexics in recovery need the support of loved ones, and this chapter offers suggestions for parents, spouses, friends, and others willing to assist.

• *Accept that there are no simple solutions.*

Eating disorders are complex illnesses. The causes are multi-faceted, and the recovery process requires self-discovery on many levels. Avoid jumping to conclusions about the how's and why's of your loved one's situation, as well as what is going to help them the most. Persevere, get educated, and realize that no single treatment approach will work for everyone. Acknowledge and honor the uniqueness of the individual you're helping.

• *Remember, anorexia is not about food.*

Beware of statements like, "If she would just eat, everything would be fine." Recovery is about revealing what lies beneath the fears related to food and weight. It is a process that demands an introspective look at one's beliefs, feelings, relationships, cultural influences, family background, etc. Gaining weight is not the only criteria for wellness, because true healing requires nourishing every aspect of the individual—mind, body and spirit.

• *Don't engage in power struggles over food.*

Your loved ones need to make their own food choices. Do not label foods as "good" or "bad" or set arbitrary rules about meals. Avoid focusing on what, how, or when they eat. However, do suggest making contracts about their eating goals. Nutritionists and dieticians can help develop a meal plan, but you should not feel responsible for making or enforcing it. If the recovering anorexic isn't meeting the agreed-upon standards, encourage her or him to honor the contract or review it with the professional who helped create it in the first place.

• *Be patient and supportive throughout the process.*

Recovery takes time and patience from everyone involved. Sometimes we worry so much about saving someone from their pain that we go to the opposite extreme and try to rush them out of it before they've had a chance to heal. Many people worry that their loved one will be trapped in that pain forever. Just being there often provides the most healing comfort available.

• *Develop open, honest lines of communication.*

You need to be able to give each other gentle feedback about the productive, and at times unproductive, things that you both do and say to each other. Listen attentively and with compassion. Don't make devaluing statements like, "Oh, don't let that bother you. It's not important." Reflective statements are much better, like, "That sounds so frustrating, I can only imagine how angry you must feel." Be non-judgemental, accepting, and willing to see things from their point-of-view. Let them know that they are not alone, that you appreciate them, and that you are trying to understand them on a deeper level.

• *You can't take away their feelings.*

Give them the space to experience their emotions. Do not try to "fix" their feelings of pain, anger, frustration, fear, etc. Nor should you expect them to immediately feel better as they work through their problems. You may feel compelled to give advice or to cheer them up, but sometimes they need to suffer. Think about a time in your life when you had an emotional crisis. You didn't want to hear, "It's not that bad," or "You should get over it." Neither do they. Remind yourself that all feelings are legitimate and serve a purpose—they need to be experienced. Offer compassion and a shoulder to cry on, and allow the tears to flow. When discussion is helpful, provide objective insight to help your loved one understand these emotions.

• *Recognize the individual separate from the eating disorder.*

Don't think of him or her as an "anorexic" but rather as someone who is "recovering from anorexia." There *is* a difference. Everyone has many characteristics and qualities, so don't concentrate only on your loved one's anorexia. Pay attention to their sense of humor, intelligence, interests, and the way they touch your heart. Encourage them to be human...not perfect.

• *Encourage him or her to seek treatment.*

Few are able to recover from anorexia alone, and professional help makes the process move more quickly and smoothly. You can offer compelling reasons for your loved one to work with therapists, doctors, nutritionists, or treatment facilities. You can also help with decisions about which options to pursue. Keep in mind that the results of treatment will be much more positive if the one in recovery makes the choices. You can help find resources, go along on appointments, pay or participate when appropriate, and be encouraging throughout therapy, but you cannot force them to do the work.

• *Recognize your own limits.*

You are not the one in recovery, so there are limits to what you can do to help. Obviously, you cannot eat for an anorexic, nor can you change another's thought patterns, beliefs, etc. In addition, they need to be responsible for their own life—from mundane activities, like getting to therapy appointments, making food choices, or cleaning up the bathroom after purging, to deeper matters, such as choosing whether to live or die. Also, you need to be clear about your personal limits regarding time, energy, and expertise. While your loved one's well-being is important to you, be careful not to deplete yourself—if you get burned out, you can't help anyone. Professional help or other support are also options for *you*.

• *Explore your own views on food, weight, and body image.*

If you are weight conscious, you are not going to help someone with anorexia feel comfortable about eating and gaining weight. After all, you are influential in this person's life; what you believe is important. Since everyone is subjected to culture's glorification of thinness, explore your own beliefs in this area. The diet mentality is harmful for most people; it can be deadly for an anorexic.

• *Do not make comments about appearance.*

Bodies come in all shapes and sizes. Concentrate on inner rather than outer beauty. Those with eating disorders tend to overanalyze anything said about their weight, so it is better for you not to talk about it at all. Even a simple statement like, "You look great," can be misinterpreted.

• *Do not speak in judgemental terms.*

Avoid making comments about other people's behavior or appearance. Reflect your own experiences by using "I" statements; "You" statements are often accusatory and diminish your loved one's personal power. For example, it is better to say, "I am worried about your weight loss," than, "You're too thin!"

* * *

Here are insights from recovered and recovering anorexics:

My father never said anything at all. He would look at me in a way that I thought was critical, and I would get so mad. We started going to family therapy, which made a big difference. I found out that he was actually worried and cared a lot; he was just afraid to say something that might make everything worse. My advice to family members is to at least tell the person that you care about them so that they don't go around thinking you don't.

If you are a family member of an anorexic, don't tell her to "eat." The problem goes deeper and isn't that easy. If she could eat normally, she would.

Having an understanding mom has been the most helpful. I explain things to her, and she really listens and tries to learn. She will sometimes offer me another point of view, but she doesn't insist that I agree with her.

When I entered therapy, my husband went with me the first couple of times and occasionally after that. We both grew a lot in the process, and our marriage became stronger as a result. He'd look me in the eye, tell me that he loved me no matter what, and made me feel more capable of recovering.

I knew that my anorexia was hard on the people I loved, but I wanted them to acknowledge that it was even harder for me.

My ex-boyfriend always told me that he liked me thin, so I felt that it was important to keep losing weight to help our relationship. That's why he's my "ex."

I really appreciated the patience of some of my friends. They asked me how they could help, and I gave them some suggestions. I told them that going out to eat was always hard for me, and the next time we went, I appreciated how supportive they were...telling me not to rush and that everything was okay.

I think one of the most helpful things in recovery was having my friends and family talk to me about things that didn't relate to food. It was nice when my best friend and I would discuss a great novel, and I enjoyed debating politics with my father. When my friends confided in me about some of the challenges that they were facing, I was reminded that I was a trustworthy person.

Resources

Non-Profit Associations

AED
Academy for Eating Disorders
Degnon Associates, Inc.
6728 Old McLean Village Dr.
McLean, VA 22101-3906
(703) 556-9222
www.acadeatdis.org
For eating disorders professionals; promotes effective treatment,
develops prevention initiatives, stimulates research, sponsors
international conference.

ANAD
National Association of Anorexia Nervosa and Associated Disorders
Box 7
Highland Park, IL 60035
(708)831-3438
www.healthtouch.com/level1/leaflets/anad/anad001.htm
Distributes listing of therapists, hospitals and informative materi-
als; sponsors support groups, conference, research, and a crisis
hot line.

EDAP
Eating Disorders Awareness and Prevention
603 Stewart St. #803
Seattle, WA 98101
(206)382-3587
members.aol.com/edapinc/home.html
Sponsors Eating Disorders Awareness Week annually in February
with a network of state coordinators and programs; distributes
educational information.

IAEDP
International Association of Eating Disorders Professionals
427 Wooping Lop #1819
Alta Monte Springs, FL 32701
(800) 800-8126
www.iaedp.com
A membership organization for professionals; provides certifica-
tion, education, local chapters, a newsletter, and an annual sym-
posium.

NEDO
National Eating Disorders Organization
6655 S. Yale Ave.
Tulsa, OK 74136
(918)481-4044
www.laureate.com/nedo-con.html
Focuses on prevention, education, research, and treatment referrals; distributes information.

Books and Internet

The Eating Disorders Resource Catalogue
PO Box 2238
Carlsbad, CA 92018
(800)756-7533
www.bulimia.com
Offers free catalogue of more than 125 books on eating disorders, non-profit associations, and treatment facilities. The Internet site includes books, links to many other eating disorders pages, lists of videos, with information about and links to treatment facilities.

Eating Disorders: A Reference Sourcebook
Edited by Ray Lemberg, Ph.D.
Oryx Press
4041 North Central at Indian School Rd.
Phoenix, AZ 85012
(602)265-6250
This book has current information about eating disorders and also includes an extensive bibliography, a list of videos, and addresses and descriptions of more than 100 inpatient treatment programs.

The Eating Disorders Sourcebook
by Carolyn Costin, M.A., M.Ed. M.F.C.C.
Lowell House/NTC
4255 West Touhy Ave.
Lincolnwood, IL 60646
(800)323-4900
This book is a comprehensive guide to eating disorders, and includes a section with addresses and descriptions of many treatment programs.

The Something Fishy Website on Eating Disorders
www.something-fishy.com
Signs and symptoms, physical dangers, definitions, words for victims sufferings, family and friends bulletin board, treatment options, a memorial page dedicated to people who have died of eating disorders, Links to other sites, chat rooms, guest speakers, and much more.

The Mirror-Mirror Website on Eating Disorders
www.mirror-mirror.org/eatdis.htm
Definitions, signs and symptoms, physical dangers, specific information on athletes, men and children with eating disorders, relapse warning signs, and much more; also has links to many web personal sites from individuals who have had or recovered from eating disorders.

Bibliography

American Psychiatric Association (APA). *Diagnostic and Statistical Manual of Mental Disorders (4th ed.)*. Washington, DC: APA, 1994.

Andersen, Arnold. "Eating Disorders in Males." in Brownell and Fairburn, 1996.

Brownell, Kelly D. and Fairburn, Christopher G., eds. *Eating Disorders and Obesity: A Comprehensive Handbook*. New York: Guilford Press, 1995.

Bruch, Hilde. *The Golden Cage: The Enigma Of Anorexia Nervosa*. New York: Vintage, 1979.

Chernin, Kim. *The Obsession: Reflections on the Tyranny of Slenderness*. New York: HarperCollins, 1981.

Bills, Eileen T. "From Sexual Abuse to Empowerment" in Hall, Lindsey. *Full Lives*, 1993.

Crisp, Arthur H., Joughin, N., Halek, C., et. al. *Anorexia Nervosa: The Wish to Change, Second Edition*. East Sussex, UK: Psychology Press, 1996.

Fodor, Viola. *Desperately Seeking Self*. Carlsbad, CA: Gürze Books, 1997.

Garner, David M. and Garfinkel, Paul E., eds. *Handbook of Treatment for Eating Disorders, Second Edition*. New York: Guilford Press, 1997.

Goodman, Charisse W. *The Invisible Woman: Confronting Weight Prejudice in America*. Carlsbad, CA: Gürze Books, 1995.

Hall, Lindsey. *Bulimia: A Guide To Recovery.* Carlsbad, CA: Gürze Books, 1992.

Hall, Lindsey. *Full Lives: Women Who Have Freed Themselves From Food & Weight Obsession.* Carlsbad, CA: Gürze Books, 1993.

Hall, Lindsey and Cohn, Leigh. *Self-Esteem Tools for Recovery.* Carlsbad, CA: Gürze Books, 1990.

Hamburg, Paul. "How Long is Long-Term Therapy for Anorexia Nervosa?" in Werne, Joellen, and Irwin D. Yallom, eds. *Treating Eating Disorders.* San Francisco: Jossey-Bass, 1996.

Kano, Susan. "Leap of Faith" in Hall, Lindsey. *Full Lives,* 1993.

Kano, Susan. *Making Peace With Food.* New York: HarperCollins, 1989.

Kaplan, Allan, and Paul Garfinkel. *Medical Issues and the Eating Disorders: The Interface.* New York: Brunner/Mazel, 1993.

Kearney-Cooke, Ann and Striegal-Moore, Ruth. "Treatment of Childhood Sexual Abuse in Anorexia Nervosa and Bulimia Nervosa: A Feminist Psychodynamic Approach" in Schwartz and Cohn, 1996.

Keys, A., Brozek, J., Henschel, A., et. al. *The Biology of Human Starvation.* Minneapolis, MN: University of Minnesota Press, 1950.

Lask, Bryan, and Rachel Bryant-Waugh. *Childhood Onset Anorexia Nervosa and Related Eating Disorders.* 1993. East Sussex, UK: Psychology Press, 1996.

Latimer, Jane. *Beyond the Food Game.* Denver, CO: LivingQuest, 1993.

Maine, Margo. *Father Hunger: Fathers, Daughters, and Food.* Carlsbad, CA: Gürze Books, 1991.

Marx, Russell. *It's Not Your Fault: Overcoming Anorexia and Bulimia Through Biopsychiatry.* New York: Plume, 1992.

Miller, Caroline Adams. "Tapestry of Recovery" in Hall, Lindsey. *Full Lives,* 1993.

Pumariega, Andres J., et. al. "Eating Attitudes in African-American Women: The *Esssence* Eating Disorders Study." *Eating Disorders: The Journal of Treatment and Prevention* 2:1, Spring 1994.

Reiff, Dan and Reiff, Kim Lampson. *Eating Disorders: Nutrition Therapy in the Recovery Process.* Englewood, CO: Aspen Publishers, 1992.

Rose, Laura. *Life Isn't Weighed on the Bathroom Scale.* Waco, TX: WRS Group, 1994.

Rubel, Jean. "Are You Finding What You Need?" in Hall, Lindsey. *Full Lives,* 1993.

Schwartz, Mark, and Leigh Cohn., eds. *Sexual Abuse and Eating Disorders.* New York: Brunner/Mazel, 1996.

Thompson, Becky. *A Hunger So Wide And So Deep.* Minneapolis: University of Minnesota Press, 1996.

Walsh, Timothy B. "Pharmacotherapy of Eating Disorders." in Brownell and Fairburn, 1995.

Yager, Joel, ed. "Anorexia Nervosa: Predicting Prognosis." *Eating Disorders Review 8:6,* 1997a.

Yager, Joel, ed. "Dexamethasone Stimulates Appetite in Anorexia Nervosa." *Eating Disorders Review* 8:3, 1997b.

Yager, Joel, ed. "What Increases the Risk of Eating Disorders Among Men?" *Eating Disorders Review* 9:2, 1998.

Zerbe, Kathryn. *The Body Betrayed: A Deeper Understanding of Women, Eating Disorders, and Treatment.* Carlsbad, CA: Gürze Books, 1995.

About the Authors

Lindsey Hall is the respected author of several books on eating disorders and recovery topics. Her best-known titles are *Bulimia: A Guide to Recovery, Self-Esteem Tools for Recovery,* and *Full Lives: Women Who Have Freed Themselves from Food & Weight Obsession,* all of which have been translated into other languages, such as French, Italian, Japanese, and Chinese. She has also edited numerous other books that have been published by Gürze Books, which she owns with her husband, Leigh Cohn. A graduate of Stanford University with a B.A. in Psychology (1971), Lindsey was the first recovered bulimic to appear on national television to share her story. She has lectured throughout the United States, served as Executive Director of Eating Disorders Awareness and Prevention, Inc., and co-founded *The Eating Disorders Resource Catalogue.* Beginning in the late '70s, Lindsey also pioneered the soft-sculpture art form, designing and selling more than a half-million Gürze dolls throughout the world. Lindsey and Leigh are the parents of two sons, Neil and Charlie.

Monika Ostroff graduated from Wellesley College in 1989 with a B.A. in Political Science. She has been active in the field of eating disorders for the past eight years. Monika has extensive experience speaking publicly and presenting workshops on etiology, treatment, and recovery from eating disorders. She has also facilitated several recovery support groups, appeared on Boston's WGBH radio Arts and Ideas educational talk show, and has authored several well-received essays on the topics of anorexia, bulimia, trauma, and healing. Today Monika continues to speak and present workshops on eating disorders, while studying for her M.S.W. degree in the clinical program at Boston College Graduate School of Social Work. She and Sam are happily married and share their home with their two cats, Faith and Cleo.

About the Publisher

Since 1980, Gürze Books has specialized in providing quality information on eating disorders recovery, research, education, advocacy, and prevention. It distributes *The Eating Disorders Resource Catalogue,* which is used as a resource throughout the world, and publishes the *Eating Disorders Review,* a clinical newsletter for professionals.

Order Form

Anorexia Nervosa: A Guide to Recovery is available at bookstores and libraries. Copies may also be ordered directly from Gürze Books.

FREE Catalogue

The Eating Disorders Resource Catalogue has more than 125 books on eating disorders and related topics, including body image, size-acceptance, self-esteem, and more. It is a valuable resource that includes listings of non-profit associations, and it is handed out by therapists, educators, and other health care professionals throughout the world.

_____ **FREE** copies of the *Eating Disorders Resource Catalogue*

_____ copies of *Anorexia Nervosa: A Guide to Recovery*
$13.95 each (1-4 copies) plus $3.00 each for shipping and handling

_____ copies of *Anorexia Nervosa: A Guide to Recovery*
$10.95 each (5+ copies) plus $2.00 each for shipping and handling

Quantity discounts are available on large orders.

NAME _____

ADDRESS _____

CITY, ST, ZIP _____

PHONE _____

Gürze Books (ANO)
P.O. Box 2238
Carlsbad, CA 92018
(760) 434-7533 • (760) 434-5476 fax
www.gurze.com